100 Questions & Answers About Your Child's Asthma

Claudia S. Plottel, MD, FACP, FCCP
New York University School of Medicine

B. Robert Feldman, MD, FAAAI, FACAAI, FAAP
Columbia College of Physicians & Surgeons/
Morgan Stanley Children's Hospital of New York-Presbyterian

JONES AND BARTLETT PUBLISHERS
Sudbury, Massachusetts
BOSTON   TORONTO   LONDON   SINGAPORE

World Headquarters
Jones and Bartlett Publishers
40 Tall Pine Drive
Sudbury, MA 01776
978-443-5000
info@jbpub.com
www.jbpub.com

Jones and Bartlett Publishers
Canada
6339 Ormindale Way
Mississauga, Ontario L5V 1J2
CANADA

Jones and Bartlett Publishers
International
Barb House, Barb Mews
London W6 7PA
UK

Jones and Bartlett's books and products are available through most bookstores and online booksellers. To contact Jones and Bartlett Publishers directly, call 800-832-0034, fax 978-443-8000, or visit our website, www.jbpub.com.

Substantial discounts on bulk quantities of Jones and Bartlett's publications are available to corporations, professional associations, and other qualified organizations. For details and specific discount information, contact the special sales department at Jones and Bartlett via the above contact information or send an email to specialsales@jbpub.com.

The authors, editor, and publisher have made every effort to provide accurate information. However, they are not responsible for errors, omissions, or for any outcomes related to the use of the contents of this book and take no responsibility for the use of the products and procedures described. Treatments and side effects described in this book may not be applicable to all people; likewise, some people may require a dose or experience a side effect that is not described herein. Drugs and medical devices are discussed that may have limited availability controlled by the Food and Drug Administration (FDA) for use only in a research study or clinical trial. Research, clinical practice, and government regulations often change the accepted standard in this field. When consideration is being given to use of any drug in the clinical setting, the health care provider or reader is responsible for determining FDA status of the drug, reading the package insert, and reviewing prescribing information for the most up-to-date recommendations on dose, precautions, and contraindications, and determining the appropriate usage for the product. This is especially important in the case of drugs that are new or seldom used.

Production Credits
Executive Publisher: Christopher Davis
Production Director: Amy Rose
Composition: Appingo
Special Projects Editor: Elizabeth Platt
Associate Editor: Kathy Richardson
Marketing Manager: Rebecca Wasley

Manufacturing and Inventory Control:
  Therese Connell
Cover Design: Jonathan Ayotte
Cover Image: © Ron Chapple 2002
  © Ilene MacDonald/Alamy Images
  © Liquid Library
Printing and Binding: Malloy, Inc.

Library of Congress Cataloging-in-Publication Data
Plottel, Claudia S.
   100 questions & answers about your child's asthma / Claudia S. Plottel, B. Robert Feldman.
      p. cm.
   Includes bibliographical references and index.
   ISBN 978-0-7637-3917-1
   1. Asthma in children—Miscellanea. I. Feldman, Bernard R. II. Title. III. Title: One hundred questions and answers about your child's asthma.
   RJ436.A8P62 2007
   618.92'238—dc22
                                        2007013968
6048

Printed in the United States of America
11 10 09 08 07   10 9 8 7 6 5 4 3 2 1

CONTENTS

The question that immediately presents itself as you thumb through *100 Questions & Answers About Your Child's Asthma* is: "Why write a book for parents about asthma in children?" One answer would revolve around numbers. We are, after all, in the midst of an asthma epidemic. The latest statistics indicate that asthma, the most common chronic disease of childhood, affects an estimated 6.5 million children in the United States. You thus probably know at least one child—perhaps a relative, a friend of your child's, or a neighborhood youngster—who has asthma. If you are the parent, family member, or caregiver of a child with asthma, you likely want to know more about pediatric asthma, understand the condition better, learn about contemporary developments, and obtain the best care for your child.

100 Questions & Answers About Your Child's Asthma reveals how far medical science has advanced in understanding asthma and how much progress we have achieved in addressing and controlling the disease in young people. New, more effective medicines have made their way into clinical practice to take their place alongside older, proven remedies. Modern asthma treatment includes more than the prescription of medications, however: there is now a greater emphasis than ever before on addressing the role that environmental factors play in asthma. Recognizing the importance of a therapeutic partnership between the child with asthma, the parents, and the treating physician is another key component of effective care for any youngster with asthma. Individualized asthma self-management programs provide a useful framework for parents and children to learn about asthma in general and to decide how asthma is best treated in their child in particular.

We are board-certified physicians who specialize in the care of infants, children, adolescents, and adults who have asthma; together, our combined practice experience exceeds sixty years. We recognize on a daily basis our obligation as physicians to provide clear and exact disease-specific information to our patients and to their families. We chose to step out of the office and the clinic to collaboratively write answers to the questions most frequently asked of us in caring for persons diagnosed with asthma. The result now lies in your hands. The one hundred questions that we selected as the backbone of *100 Questions & Answers About Your Child's Asthma* are real questions, ones we find ourselves answering again and again in our professional lives. The format of the book mirrors the sequence of a medical consultation, but the question-and-answer format allows you to flip through the book and read ahead to those topics that most interest you, in any order you prefer. We have included a listing of asthma resources for further reading after Question 100 and have composed a glossary of important vocabulary terms to facilitate your reading and understanding.

100 Questions & Answers About Your Child's Asthma provides scientific, accurate, and timely information that reflects both the medical profession's current understanding of asthma and our own experience as practicing asthma specialists. It also incorporates the experiences of people who have seen pediatric asthma up close. Frank Lomascolo, now a college student, has carried a diagnosis of asthma since childhood, and Kerrin Robinson is the mother of a toddler with asthma. Both have most generously offered their complementary yet honest perspectives on living with asthma. Their unique contributions to our book significantly enhance its value and usefulness. We wish to acknowledge Christopher Davis, Executive Publisher for Medicine at Jones and Bartlett Publishers, who has been steadfast in his support for *100 Questions & Answers About Your Child's Asthma*. We are especially grateful to Elizabeth Platt, Special Projects Editor at Jones and Bartlett Publishers, for her enthusiasm about our project, her professionalism, her top-notch editorial expertise, and not least, her unfailing good humor. We have greatly enjoyed writing the book you now have before you. It has made us think about how best to communicate medical information and how to present the "doctor's side" of asthma while striking a balance between complex scientific information and everyday practicalities. We hope that you will learn as much from reading *100 Questions & Answers About Your Child's Asthma* as we did from writing it.

Claudia S. Plottel, MD, FACP, FCCP
B. Robert Feldman, MD, FAAAI, FACAAI, FAAP
New York City

ACKNOWLEDGMENTS

To my husband, Larry Stam, MD, who with Elisabeth and Charles Stam consistently encouraged my efforts and listened to my ramblings about sentence structure and grammatical construction: thank you from the bottom of my heart.

—*Claudia S. Plottel*

To my wife, Clare, who has been my constant source of encouragement for the past 46 years; my son, David, whose assistance as a critic and my techno-advisor has played an invaluable role in the production of this book; and to my daughter, Janet, who never stops telling me that "I'm the best"—you have my never-ending love.

—*B. Robert Feldman*

Dedication

For Charles and for Elisabeth.
Love you always, now and forever . . .
CSP

To all the patients I have cared for who never
stop asking questions, this book will hopefully
provide you with some of the answers.
BRF

PART ONE

General Information

What is asthma?

What causes asthma?

Why is asthma so common?

Do more boys than girls have asthma?

What are asthma triggers?

More . . .

Asthma

A chronic respiratory condition characterized by breathing symptoms of varying intensity and frequency. Asthma has a strong genetic (inherited) basis, although environmental influences also play an important role. Asthma frequently goes hand-in-hand with allergy, especially in younger age groups.

Chronic

Longstanding, lingering, or expected to last indefinitely.

Bronchial passageways

The breathing tubes of the lungs.

Mucus

A mixture composed of water, salt, and proteins produced by specialized cells in the nose, sinuses, and lung passages. Mucus plays a defensive role and helps to protect against infection.

Asthma is a chronic disease that involves the bronchial passageways, which are the breathing tubes of the lungs.

1. What is asthma?

Asthma is the most common chronic disease of childhood. Asthma affects all age groups. It can manifest itself throughout childhood, from infancy to late adolescence and even beyond. Asthma is a lung disease that involves the lungs' airways or breathing tubes. In a large number of children, an allergic tendency often accompanies asthma. Asthma is best defined as a physical condition involving the lungs, a pulmonary disease targeting bronchial passageways, which are the breathing tubes of the lungs.

Asthma is characterized from a patient's perspective by symptoms of varying intensity and frequency. Asthma symptoms are related to the lungs and to breathing. Typical symptoms of asthma include intermittent cough, mucus production, wheezing, along with breathlessness and "uncomfortable" breathing with sensations of chest tightness or pressure. Some children have very mild asthma and may experience few or no symptoms for much of the year. Others at the opposite end of the asthma spectrum may regularly require several medications every day to normalize their lung function and attain a symptom-free state.

We strongly believe that participation in a comprehensive medical management program is crucial to a favorable asthma outcome. Part of successful asthma treatment includes learning about asthma and mastering self-management skills. In particular, the development of close and effective working relationships between parents and the health care team is a critical component of the overall treatment program and ensures the best possible care for any child with asthma. With proper medical care and three-way cooperation among patient, parents, and the treating physician, a child diagnosed with asthma can look forward to a full and satisfying life (Table 1).

Table 1 Asthma Facts

Children (and adults) can die from poorly controlled asthma.
Participation in sports and regular exercise is encouraged and is part of a comprehensive asthma treatment plan for all ages.
Maintenance of physical fitness is an integral part of asthma management.
A critically important aspect of optimal asthma control is the reduction and potential elimination of inflammation within the lungs.
Elimination of wheezing and breathlessness is a major asthma treatment goal.
Obesity is associated with asthma.
Asthma has a genetic basis and somtimes occurs or "runs" in familes.
Asthma and allergy have a strong correlation in children, and they often coexist and overlap.
It is common for asthma to seemingly "disappear" during adolescence, but many teenagers will experience re-emergence of their asthma years later, in adulthood.
The majority of children who experience asthma symptoms through their teenage years will likely continue with this condition as adults.

2. How do lungs work and function?

The lungs are part of the respiratory system (Figure 1). The lungs take oxygen (O_2) into the body and rid it of accumulated carbon dioxide (CO_2). A good way to understand the workings of the lungs is to first get an overview of their structure, or anatomy (Figure 1A). The human respiratory system begins at the nose and includes the nasal passages, which warm, humidify, and filter inhaled air as it travels past the throat and enters the windpipe, or trachea. The trachea sits below the voice box (larynx). Its uppermost portion can be felt in the front of the neck as it descends behind the breastbone (sternum) into the chest. The trachea then divides into two branches: the right mainstem bronchus and the left mainstem bronchus. The right mainstem bronchus leads air to and from the right lung, and the left mainstem bronchus leads air to and from the left lung. The right lung is larger than the left;

General Information

Carbon dioxide

An odorless, colorless gas produced as a by-product of the body's metabolism; it is normally excreted by the lungs.

Trachea

The scientific name for the windpipe. The uppermost portion of the trachea can be felt in the front of the neck. The trachea leads air from the back of the nose and throat into the lungs.

Larynx

The voice box. Two vocal cords allow for speech as inhaled air passes between them and creates vibrations within the larynx located in the mid-neck.

Bronchus (pl. bronchi)

A lung breathing passage or tube.

A **Lung Anatomy**

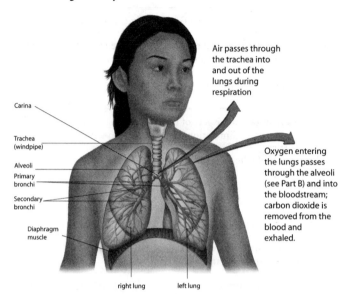

Air passes through the trachea into and out of the lungs during respiration

Oxygen entering the lungs passes through the alveoli (see Part B) and into the bloodstream; carbon dioxide is removed from the blood and exhaled.

Carina

Trachea (windpipe)

Alveoli

Primary bronchi

Secondary bronchi

Diaphragm muscle

right lung   left lung

B **Respiration: The Process of Breathing**

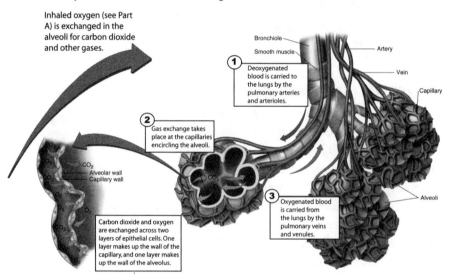

Inhaled oxygen (see Part A) is exchanged in the alveoli for carbon dioxide and other gases.

Bronchiole

Smooth muscle

Artery

Vein

Capillary

1 Deoxygenated blood is carried to the lungs by the pulmonary arteries and arterioles.

2 Gas exchange takes place at the capillaries encircling the alveoli.

Alveolar wall
Capillary wall

Carbon dioxide and oxygen are exchanged across two layers of epithelial cells. One layer makes up the wall of the capillary, and one layer makes up the wall of the alveolus.

3 Oxygenated blood is carried from the lungs by the pulmonary veins and venules.

Alveoli

remember that the heart is located in the left chest, and therefore the left lung is smaller than the right to make room for the heart. The right side of the chest, on the other hand, only contains the right lung.

The point at which the trachea divides into the right and left mainstem bronchi is called the carina. After the split, the right and left mainstem bronchi each lead to their respective lung and subdivide into smaller and smaller tube-like passages, creating the branching tracheobronchial tree. As the bronchi continue to subdivide into successively narrower bronchi, they ultimately end in the tiniest subdivision, the bronchiole. Each bronchiole leads to the air sacs, the alveoli.

The alveoli are specialized lung structures. They allow fresh oxygen-rich inhaled air to enter the body and oxygen-poor, carbon dioxide–rich air to exit (Figure 1B). Oxygen is required for life, and therefore oxygen deprivation is rapidly fatal. As oxygen enters the bloodstream and is transported to all organs, the "used" air, now composed mostly of carbon dioxide, is removed from the body (or "excreted") by exhalation. Carbon dioxide is produced by the body's metabolism, and is considered a metabolic waste product.

Abnormal accumulation of carbon dioxide in the body and in the bloodstream is detrimental to health and is seen in certain forms of respiratory failure. The process responsible for the body's oxygen uptake and its carbon dioxide removal (or excretion) is called respiration. Respiration is the primary, crucial function of the lungs and respiratory system. Physicians may refer to respiration as gas exchange. Gas exchange occurs in the deepest portion of the lung, at the level of the alveoli. Oxygen and carbon dioxide exchange occurs along a specialized zone where each air sac (alveolus) is in intimate contact with tiny blood vessels called capillaries. The capillary bed completely encircles the alveoli along the alveolar-capillary membrane. When respiration is impaired, blood

Carina

The split where the trachea divides into two branches: the right mainstem bronchus and the left mainstem bronchus. Each bronchus leads air to the right and left lung respectively.

Bronchiole

The fine, tapered, thin-walled breathing passages that branch and extend from the bronchi and end in the alveolar air sacs.

Alveoli

Air sacs in the lung where oxygen is exchanged for carbon dioxide (*see alveolus*). A healthy adult human lung contains approximately 300 million alveoli.

General Information

oxygen levels may decrease as carbon dioxide levels rise and acids build up in the body. If the abnormal accumulation of acid and carbon dioxide is not corrected, respiratory failure, a potentially life-threatening condition, will develop. Although uncontrolled asthma can lead to respiratory failure and death, as discussed in Question 20, it is a rare complication.

3. Do lungs continue to develop after birth?

Yes. Lungs continue to grow and develop after a normal, term pregnancy. The specialized gas-exchanging lung units called alveoli, where oxygen is exchanged for carbon dioxide, develop postnatally. In fact, nearly 85% of the lung alveoli are formed after birth during the first three years of life. The blood supply within the capillary network matures along with alveolar development from birth to 3 years of age. Mucus-producing lung cells also develop after birth.

Because most alveoli develop postnatally, the first three years of life can be viewed as an especially vulnerable period. In the era before antibiotics, young children who became afflicted with bacterial pneumonia or tuberculosis during alveolar development and survived the infection were left with pulmonary impairment. The introduction of antibiotic and antituberculous medicines after World War II unquestionably reduced the number and severity of damaging lung infections in children. Children growing up today face a different but nonetheless very serious and all-too-prevalent obstacle to normal lung maturation: cigarettes and tobacco. Secondary smoke (or as lung specialists call it, environmental tobacco smoke, or ETS) has been designated a Group A carcinogen or cancer-causing agent by the U.S. Environmental Protection Agency. The Group A carcinogen classification is reserved for only the most dangerous cancer-causing agents in humans. In addition to being a confirmed carcinogen, ETS adversely affects the lungs of growing children. Scientific data clearly and unequivocally show that exposure to ETS, or second-hand smoke, leads to at least six significant adverse health effects in children, and that three of these ill effects involve the lungs. Children exposed to ETS experience an increased frequency of acute lower respiratory tract infections, persistent chronic respiratory symptoms (e.g., cough), and are at a significantly higher risk for developing asthma and subsequent recurring asthma exacerbations. The extra-respiratory effects of childhood ETS exposure include delivery of low birth weight babies, a higher risk for sudden infant death syndrome (SIDS), and an increased number of middle ear infections in childhood.

After the age of three, the lungs are basically formed but not yet fully developed. As the body continues to mature from adolescence to adulthood, so do the lungs. The period of adolescence represents a second window of lung vulnerability. Recent scientific studies indicate that teenagers who smoke cigarettes will end up with lung function that is less than expected; their lungs will never attain their predicted level of function. The finding of stunted lung function development in adolescent smokers is especially notable in girls.

4. What causes asthma?

Asthma has no single, easily identifiable cause. The interaction of several different factors seems to be necessary for a child to develop the disease. Studies have shown that asthma often runs in certain families. The tendency to develop asthma clearly has a genetic basis. Children born to parents with asthma have an increased risk of developing asthma as compared to children of nonasthmatic parents. Similarly, a child's risk of developing allergies is increased if either parent carries a diagnosis of allergy. The connection seems to be more powerful if the mother rather than the father has allergies and/or asthma. A study of 344 families residing in Arizona showed that among children with asthma, only 6% were from families in which neither parent had asthma, 20% had one parent with asthma, and 60% had two parents with asthma.

General Information

Alveolus (pl. alveoli)

A lung's air sac. Oxygen is exchanged for carbon dioxide in the lung alveoli. A dense network of capillary vessels surrounds each alveolus. The close arrangement allows for very rapid exchange (or diffusion) of oxygen from alveolus to capillary, and of carbon dioxide from capillary to alveolus.

Capillary

A tiny thin-walled blood vessel. The lungs' capillaries play a crucial role in health as part of the alveolar–capillary membrane, absorbing oxygen into the body and getting rid of carbon dioxide.

Postnatally

After birth. Human lungs continue to grow and develop postnatally, after birth and into infancy.

The interaction of several different factors may be necessary for a child to develop asthma.

Chromosome

A microscopic structure with groupings of DNA that contain many genes, regulatory elements, and other intervening nucleotide DNA sequences, found in the nucleus of all human cells. Humans normally have 23 pairs of chromosomes.

Molecular biology

The study of the structure, function, and reactions of DNA, RNA, proteins, and other molecules involved in the life processes.

Data from studies of asthma and allergy in identical and fraternal twins show an inherited basis for the development of asthma. The actual detailed mode of inheritance is not yet known. Much research is under way worldwide to identify the specific genes that are responsible for asthma. Investigation involving several genes on different chromosomes has so far produced data indicating that no one single asthma gene exists. Current thinking is that several separate asthma genes interact to produce the clinical symptoms that we recognize as bronchial asthma. The theory further suggests that specific environmental exposures, must at some point, interact with susceptibility genes to produce clinical symptoms. Advances in molecular biology will hopefully not only lead to the identification of specific asthma genes but also identify the genes responsible for disease severity (such as asthma severity–modifying genes).

Asthma often coexists with a diagnosis of allergy, especially in children and in teenagers. Asthma similarly occurs very commonly in children who also have allergic rhinitis. Clinicians who treat both adults and children have long noted that certain viral infections seem to be related to the development of asthma in predisposed individuals. Physicians, for example, describe "asthmagenic" viruses that cause typical respiratory infection and symptoms at first, only to leave the patient with an asthma-like medical condition after all the initial respiratory symptoms have resolved.

The above observations, along with a large body of research findings, have led to the current view that asthma is probably caused by a complex interaction between a susceptible individual and certain environmental conditions (Figure 2).

Possible Environmental Factors in Asthma Development

The development of asthma reflects a particular genetic or innate predisposition to the disease. In addition, environmental influences have been recognized as significant in the emergence of clinical asthma. The precise interplay between environmental and hereditary factors leading to asthma is still insufficiently understood. It is has long been noted that some environmental exposures are associated with progression to asthma while other types of exposure might possibly prevent or delay the development of asthma in susceptible persons. The complex relationships are the subject of ongoing research, at the molecular level, in laboratory animals, and in human populations.

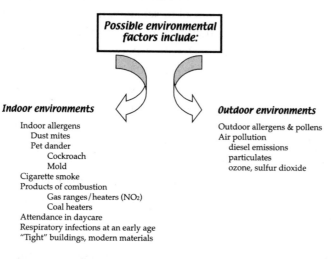

Possible environmental factors include:

Indoor environments

Indoor allergens
  Dust mites
  Pet dander
    Cockroach
    Mold
Cigarette smoke
Products of combustion
    Gas ranges/heaters (NO₂)
    Coal heaters
Attendance in daycare
Respiratory infections at an early age
"Tight" buildings, modern materials

Outdoor environments

Outdoor allergens & pollens
Air pollution
  diesel emissions
  particulates
  ozone, sulfur dioxide

Indoor environments play a greater role than outdoor ones in terms of asthma development.

The 2000 report on: *Clearing the Air: Asthma and Indoor Air Exposures* from the Institute of Medicine concludes that there is sufficient evidence to support a causal relationship between asthma development and exposures to house dust mite (increased risk of asthma), environmental tobacco (probably increased risk). Cockroach, cat and dog carry a "maybe" increased risk.

Figure 2   Possible environmental factors in asthma development.

5. Is asthma inherited?

Yes, the tendency to develop asthma is inherited to some degree. Allergy and asthma have been noted to occur in successive generations of a single family. The precise role of human genetics and its relation to a specific medical condition, such as bronchial asthma, is a highly complex subject. There is intense interest on the part of geneticists and other medical scientists in identifying exactly which genes play a role

If a child has a family history of allergy or asthma, and particularly if the mother has asthma, there is an increased probability that the child will develop the same condition.

There is intense interest on the part of geneticists and other medical scientists in identifying exactly which genes are responsible for each and every disease.

in directly causing or in modifying the severity of specific human diseases.

The U.S. Human Genome Project is a genetic research endeavor, which began formally in 1990, took thirteen years to complete, and was coordinated by the U.S. Department of Energy and the National Institutes of Health. The project, completed two years ahead of schedule in 2003, met several goals, including the identification and localization of all the genes in human DNA. Details of the project are available at: http://www.ornl.gov/sci/techresources/Human_Genome/home.html. By completely mapping out the genes found on each human chromosome, the genome project opened the door to investigations of illnesses at the most basic, chemical level. Ongoing research continues in an attempt to pinpoint which specific genes are responsible for the development of bronchial asthma. Experts know that more than one gene is involved in transmitting the condition from one generation to the next.

Modern techniques of genetic DNA analysis might thus, in the not too distant future, provide scientists with the tools and ability to determine to what extent an individual child may be at an increased risk for developing asthma over the course of a lifetime. The hope is that when the genes responsible for asthma are clearly identified, physicians will be able to modify (or hopefully even eliminate) a child's potential for developing asthma.

6. Is asthma contagious? Can you catch asthma from someone who has it?

The answer is: no, you cannot catch asthma. Asthma is not contagious; it cannot be transmitted from person to person. Remember that there is an inherited component to the development of asthma and allergy. If one parent has asthma or is allergic, a child has a greater chance of developing asthma and/or allergies as compared to another child whose parents have neither asthma nor allergy. The chance of a child developing asthma further increases when both parents are affected. The exact role of genetics and the inheritance patterns of asthma are not well understood, and genetic inheritance alone is far from the whole story. Environmental factors clearly play a large role in asthma development. If your child has asthma, and you are later diagnosed with the same condition, this does not mean that you somehow "caught asthma" from your child; rather, your asthma diagnosis reflects genetic and environmental factors common to both you and your child.

Asthma is a medical condition that also cannot truly be "cured," a fact discussed in Question 22 as the state of bronchial hyperreactivity, inherent to asthma, persists throughout life. Asthma is however a disease that can be effectively controlled through appropriate medical care that includes patient and parental education. A child with asthma can realistically expect a full, healthy, and active lifestyle when he and his parents obtain sound medical advice, faithfully follow treatment recommendations, and forge a strong therapeutic alliance with the treating physician.

Parents often inquire whether their child will outgrow asthma, a point reviewed in detail in Question 21. Many general pediatricians falsely reassure parents that their child will outgrow their asthma by young adulthood. In fact, the physician's response should more realistically be: "I don't know." Is it possible for some asthma patients to "lose" their symptoms and reach a point where they no longer require any medication? Based on population studies, the answer is yes, the phenomenon does occur. This is a very difficult question to answer for any individual child; however, information about the family history of allergy or asthma, the age at which the child's chest symptoms first appeared, and the child's specific triggers, such as respiratory tract infections, may provide clues

*Some informa-
tion about the
family history
of allergy or
of asthma, the
age at which
the child's chest
symptoms first
appeared, and
specific trig-
gers, such as
respiratory tract
infections, may
provide clues
as to a child's
potential to
develop long-
standing, or
chronic, asthma.*

Asymptomatic

Without any manifestations or symptoms of disease or illness. The major goal of asthma treatment is to achieve an asymp-tomatic state so that the person with asthma experiences no symptoms and is able to lead a full and productive life.

Epidemiologic studies

Based on the study of populations or large groups of people.

relating to a child's potential to develop more longstanding, or chronic, asthma.

There seems to be a greater likelihood that a child will stop experiencing asthma symptoms with the passage of time if (1) they have no family history of asthma, (2) their symptoms of cough or wheezing began early in life, and (3) their primary trigger was a respiratory tract infection. Many children with these characteristics are free of asthma symptoms within the first decade of life. Other children, however, experience gradu-ally fewer and fewer asthma symptoms as they get older and then become asymptomatic during their adolescent years. It is during this time that pediatricians sometimes comment that a teenager "seems to have outgrown" his or her asthma. These young people often present to adult lung specialists many years later, well after they have "graduated" from the pedia-tricians care, and are re-diagnosed with asthma! The bottom line: a significant proportion of children who have asthma will continue to have some asthma symptoms throughout their lives, often in spite of a prolonged symptom-free interval in adolescence.

7. Is there anything I can do to prevent my child from developing asthma?

Medical science has no intervention at the present time that can prevent the asthma from affecting a given child. Because asthma tends to run in families however, physicians sometimes make suggestions to try to minimize or delay the development of allergy and asthma symptoms in a child believed to be at increased risk for the disease (Table 2). Based on epidemio-logic studies, physicians may advise expectant parents who have positive asthma histories to follow special guidelines in caring for their newborn. Many recommendations concern the baby's diet and environment. For example, an exclusive diet of mother's milk for at least the first six months of life may possibly delay the development of allergy and asthma, and certain highly allergenic foods should not be part of a toddler's diet. Several foods are responsible for most food allergy in young children. More specifically, 90% of all allergic reactions to food are caused by eight foods: cow's milk, egg, peanut (which is a legume, not a true nut), tree nuts (such as walnuts, cashews, and hazelnuts), fish, shellfish, soy, and wheat. In addition to dietary guidelines, physicians stress the importance of a 100% smoke-free home. Some doctors may advise additional environmental measures, such as ensuring that your child's bedroom's is free of dust-collecting items, such as draperies, stuffed animals, and wall-to-wall carpeting, or encasing your child's mattress in specialized covers to reduce exposure to dust mites.

Remember, parents and children with asthma are not "responsible" for "causing" their asthma to develop in the first place. Medical care today focuses on the prevention of symptoms and on keeping the condition quiescent. Research focuses on studying asthma at the level of molecular biology. By understanding more about the mechanisms of asthma itself, and by investigating what factors cause, delay, or block its development in children and adults, we will hopefully then be better able to gain insight into the root causes of asthma. Currently, there is no known way to completely prevent the development of asthma.

Dust mites

Microscopic living organisms found indoors in tempered climates, especially in mattresses, bedding, and upholstered furniture. Dust mites are a common cause of allergy and asthma exacerbation, but their numbers can be greatly reduced or nearly eliminated by control measures in the home.

Table 2 Asthma Risk Factors: Possible Hints to Causes of Asthma

Risk factors for developing asthma include:

Exposure to inhalant indoor allergens: dust mite, cockroach, cat, dog

Family history of allergy (especially in mother)

Family history of asthma (especially in mother)

Exposure to cigarette smoke

History of low birth weight

History of respiratory infections

Urbanization* (perhaps)

Urbanization seems to be associated with an increase in asthma; it is unclear if this is a separate risk or simply a reflection of increased exposure to indoor allergens. Indoor allergens are more common and concentrated in urbanized settings, especially in economically disadvantaged areas of major large cities.

Kerrin's comment:

From infancy, my son experienced allergic symptoms. He developed eczema when he was a few months old and would occasionally get hives after he breast-fed. He later experienced breathing problems that on three separate occasions escalated to the point where he needed to be hospitalized for around-the-clock breathing treatments. When he was about 2 years old, he was officially diagnosed with asthma. Knowing this, and that he had allergic tendencies but not knowing exactly what they were yet, we decided to keep him away from the highly allergenic foods, such as peanuts and cow's milk. As he got older, we would give him small portions of milk to see if he could tolerate it and he seemed to be fine. Because peanuts are the next hardest ingredient to avoid, we decided that we would have him tested for this allergy. Before we even got the chance, he took a bite of a cookie that had either been baked with peanut oil or had touched another item that contained peanut, and he shortly thereafter developed terrible hives. We immediately took him to see a pediatric allergy specialist, who tested him for peanuts and, sure enough, he had a severe allergy. We were told that the next time he is exposed to peanut, the symptoms could be even more severe and lead to compromised breathing.

8. What is the contemporary view of asthma, and how does it differ from traditional views?

Asthma is a condition that has affected humans for centuries, certainly since antiquity. The Ebers papyrus records prescriptions for asthma written in hieroglyphics! The 12th-century physician Moses Maimonides in his role as physician to the court of Saladin wrote a detailed treatise on asthma for his royal patient, Prince Al-Afdal. Incidentally, one of his recommendations was to drink soup prepared from fat hens: chicken soup!

For much of the 20th Century, asthma was viewed as a disease of airway narrowing, or bronchoconstriction. In this traditional view, the bronchial passages, especially those encircled by specialized muscle fibers, became narrowed or constricted and an inevitable attack would follow. The traditional explanation emphasized that constriction of the bronchial tubes was the major abnormal phenomenon in asthma. The focus of asthma treatment centered on attempts to reverse bronchial constriction. Consequently, treatment consisted mostly of relief of airway narrowing once asthma symptoms had developed and had become obvious. Emphasis was placed on treating attack symptoms rather than on preventive measures.

The contemporary perspective on asthma recognizes the importance of bronchoconstriction, but assigns it a secondary role. The principal "player" or "culprit" in asthma is inflammation. In the contemporary model of asthma, people with asthma experience periods of active, inadequately controlled disease or exacerbation, along with quiescent periods of good asthma control. During an exacerbation, there is increased inflammatory activity in the asthmatic lung. The inflammation, if unchecked, leads to two consequences: (1) mucus-

Broncho-constriction

An abnormal narrowing of the air passages. Bronchoconstriction is a prominent characteristic of asthma and is caused by an increased inflammatory response in the lung.

Constriction

Narrowing; the opposite of dilatation. *See also bronchoconstriction.*

Hyperreactivity

With respect to asthma, refers to asthmatic lungs' greater sensitivity to inhaled substances that would produce no symptoms in a healthy person without asthma.

Methacholine challenge test

The methacholine challenge test is a type of bronchoprovocation test. It is a specialized pulmonary function test used in evaluating suspected asthma when the diagnosis is otherwise uncertain. Methacholine challenge testing can identify bronchial hyperreactivity.

Broncho-provocation test

A specialized pulmonary function test that assesses for the presence of baseline hyperreactivity and that can be helpful in the diagnostic evaluation of suspected asthma. Both methacholine challenge testing and cold-air exercise challenge are examples of bronchoprovocation tests.

gland stimulation with excess secretions, and (2) eventual bronchoconstriction or airway narrowing. Mucus-producing glands are normal structures located in the bronchial passages. Asthmatic inflammation causes the glands to make increased amounts of mucus that are then released into the bronchial passages. The mucus thus secreted in active asthma tends to be thick and "sticky." The body's natural response is to try to expel the mucus from the bronchial tubes, by coughing it out. The increased mucus production in active asthma leads to cough. The bronchoconstriction is responsible for symptoms of chest tightness, breathlessness, uncomfortable breathing, and wheezing.

Individuals with even mild asthma, both children and adults, have been shown to develop increased inflammatory reactivity in their lungs. They are described as having increased bronchial hyperreactivity or "twitchy bronchi." A specialized pulmonary function test, called the methacholine challenge or bronchoprovocation test, is helpful to clinicians when evaluating teens and adults suspected of having bronchial hyperreactivity. The tendency toward increased baseline hyperreactivity is likely hereditary. Increased hyperreactivity explains why, for example, people with asthma are more sensitive to inhalation of different environmental stimuli, such as cold air, allergens, strong odors, or cigarette smoke. The presence of bronchial hyperreactivity is of great interest to asthma researchers. It is tempting to speculate about a medication that could modify a person's bronchial hyperreactivity, thereby reducing the severity of their asthma.

The current understanding of asthma as a disease primarily of inflammation, with secondary airway narrowing and constriction as consequences of an increased inflammatory response, has both research and practical implications. It allows for preventive interventions and more directed medications. Controlling and limiting airway inflammation reduces asthma symptoms, normalizes lung function, offers an excellent prognosis, and leads to a healthy lifestyle. Prompt treatment of an exacerbation should include anti-inflammatory treatment in addition to specific treatment of bronchoconstriction. Recognition of the importance of inflammation in asthma has led to a better understanding of asthma and to the development of more effective treatment.

Asthma exacerbations can sometimes predictably occur under certain circumstances, such as with major changes in the weather and the onset of the heating season. Some individuals, for example, experience an "attack" in the spring and fall at the change of season. Such asthma symptoms may be triggered because of an allergy to trees or grass pollen. Treatment of "an attack" in the traditional view might include increasing doses of inhaled medications or even a burst of steroid medications, ideally administered in an office or clinic setting, but possibly in an emergency department or hospital. Treatment regimens today concentrate on anti-inflammatory medications along with bronchodilators and focus on an individual child's symptom triggers and patterns of asthma exacerbations.

The contemporary view of asthma thus emphasizes a preventative approach (Table 3). A child with asthma who experiences a pattern of worsening symptoms in winter weather would be prescribed anti-inflammatory medication in the early fall, for example. The youngster whose asthma symptoms flare when trees are in bloom could similarly begin taking additional, stepped-up asthma treatments in March or April. By successfully controlling inflammation, and by being alert to early signs and symptoms of disease exacerbation, "attacks" can be averted and significant lifestyle disruptions avoided.

Recognition of the importance of inflammation in asthma has led to a better understanding of asthma and to the development of more effective treatment.

Allergen

An agent that is able to produce an abnormal (allergic) response in a susceptible individual when that person becomes exposed to the agent. An allergen is usually a protein and can be of varied origin. Specific examples of common allergens include peanut, penicillin, ragweed, and cat dander. Allergens may be asthma triggers for certain children who have both asthma and allergy.

General Information

Table 3   The Contemporary View of Asthma

The modern view of asthma emphasizes the all-important role of inflammation. Consequently, contemporary asthma treatment includes:

Using measurements of lung function
  • To assess the severity of a child's asthma
  • To follow a child's response to therapy over time

Avoiding factors that increase lung inflammation and that precipitate asthma symptoms
  • Avoiding triggers
  • Instituting environmental control measures
  • Keeping immunizations up to date

Patient and parental education
  • To create an effective partnership between the patient and the treating physician
  • To teach and refine a child's asthma self-management skills

---

Comprehensive pharmacological therapy
  • Medications are designed to reverse airway inflammation
  • Medications are designed to prevent airway inflammation
  • Medications are designed to manage symptoms and exacerbations

---

9. How many American children have asthma?

Asthma occurs in all age groups and can be diagnosed at any age, from the toddler years well into an individual's 70s or even 80s. Asthma currently affects more than 20.5 million Americans, including over 6.5 million children younger than 18 years of age. It is the primary cause of school absences from a chronic condition, with 14.7 million school days missed annually because of childhood asthma.

Exacerbation

A flare of disease activity or disease symptoms. An exacerbation of asthma leads to increased symptoms of cough, mucus, chest tightness, and wheezing.

A detailed snapshot of asthma in America in 2003 revealed that about 30 million Americans had been diagnosed with asthma by a physician at some time during their life and, of that total number, almost 20 million had active disease at the time of the survey. Another third, or 11 million individuals, had experienced an asthma exacerbation or attack in the past twelve months. The finding that a significant number of people who are diagnosed with asthma can go for twelve months without experiencing an attack reflects that (1) asthma has a range of severity, from very mild to life-threatening, and that (2) very safe and effective asthma treatments, when prescribed appropriately and taken as directed, can lead to an excellent quality of life.

The National Center for Health Statistics at the Centers for Disease Control and Prevention (CDC) estimates that in 2002, asthma in all age groups accounted for 12.7 million visits to office-based physicians, 1.2 million visits to hospital clinics, and 1.9 million emergency department visits. The same calendar year saw 484,000 hospitalizations for treatment of asthma and 4,261 deaths from asthma, with most, but not all, occurring among the adult population (Table 4). This last statistic is especially shocking because it indicates that on average, almost a dozen individuals die from asthma each day in the Unites States. Furthermore, these deaths occur at a time when science has made enormous strides in the understanding of asthma and allergy, and when safe and effective treatments have become well accepted by the medical profession. From a global perspective, asthma is responsible for about one in every two hundred fifty deaths worldwide. Asthma specialists believe that many asthma deaths could be prevented with optimal long-term medical care, patient education, and access to emergency care for treatment of an exacerbation of the disease.

Allergy

The body's physical reaction to certain external substances that involves the body's production of a specific antibody in direct response to a specific allergen. The result of the allergy–antibody interaction includes inflammatory and immune changes that, in turn, lead to symptoms potentially affecting the eyes, nose, sinuses, skin, and lungs.

Table 4   Asthma in the United States: Facts

Asthma is the most common chronic disease of childhood.

Asthma accounts for approximately 14 million lost days of school every year.

Asthma affects approximately 6.5 million children younger than 18 years.

In the year 2002, asthma accounted for 12.7 million visits to physicians' offices, 1.2 million visits to hospital clinics, and 1.9 million emergency department visits.

There were 484,000 hospitalizations for treatment of asthma in 2002.

Asthma is the third ranking cause of hospitalization among children younger than 15 years of age.

There were 4,261 deaths from asthma reported in 2002.

The number of children dying from asthma increased nearly threefold from 1980 to 1998, but since 1999 has decreased from 3.2 deaths per 1 million children to 2.5 deaths per 1 million children in 2004.

Total asthma-related health costs are estimated at $14 billion annually.

Estimated cost of treating asthma in children and adolescents younger than 18 years of age is $3.2 billion annually.

General Information

In August 2005, the CDC published its analysis of data from the 2003 national Youth Risk Behavior Survey (YRBS) in order to assess self-reported asthma and asthma attacks among American high school students. The statistics showed that 18.9% of high school students had been told by a doctor or nurse that they had asthma; nearly one in six students, or 16.1%, had current asthma; and 37.9% of those with current asthma had experienced an episode of asthma or an asthma attack during the twelve months preceding the survey. The data failed to confirm other studies' findings of differences between Caucasian and African-American high school students reporting current asthma or experiencing an asthma exacerbation in the prior twelve months. Those earlier studies had reported: (1) higher asthma prevalence among African-American children as compared with Caucasian children, and (2) that African-American children were more than three times as likely as Caucasian children to be hospitalized because of asthma and more than four times as likely to die of asthma. The YRBS results, however, indicated no difference between the percentages of African-American and Caucasian students enrolled in high school reporting current asthma or experiencing an asthma exacerbation in the prior twelve months. Interestingly, the YRBS high school data indicated that there were significantly more female students with asthma than male high school students with asthma. It also showed that significantly more students with asthma in ninth grade reported an exacerbation in the prior twelve months compared with those in tenth, eleventh, or twelfth grades.

Prevalence

In medicine, the total number of cases of a disease diagnosed at a given point in time. It includes all cases, whether the diagnosis is new or longstanding. To assess the prevalence of asthma in a community as of January 1, for example, you would count all persons who were ever told by a medical professional that they had a diagnosis of asthma.

10. Why is asthma so common?

Asthma is very common, affecting approximately one of every ten Americans at some point in their life, according to 2001 data from the Centers for Disease Control and Prevention's National Health Interview Survey. It is not clear why asthma has become such a prevalent chronic condition. One theory is that physicians have become more adept at diagnosing asthma correctly so that more cases are properly identified, and therefore better diagnosis and more accurate "counting" of cases is actually responsible for what seems to be increased prevalence of asthma. Actually, the opposite is true: the diagnosis of asthma is too often overlooked, particularly in older age groups and in adolescents, and especially in teenaged girls. The fact is that asthma has truly become more common. A more likely theory implicates various environmental factors. Smoking, for example, became socially acceptable for women after World War II. Infants of mothers who smoke have an increased risk for developing asthma during childhood. Increasing air pollutants and particulates found in urban or industrial areas may also contribute to the upswing in asthma cases. From the perspective of an asthma specialist, the enactment of laws banning smoking in all indoor public places, such as those in New York City, is a crucial step toward improving air quality.

11. Why does asthma seem to be increasing?

Asthma is unquestionably on the upswing in the United States and other industrialized nations, such as Australia and Great Britain. In 1998, for example, the Centers for Disease Control and Prevention (CDC) reported on the morbidity and mortality related to asthma in the United States between 1960 and 1995. The data showed several disconcerting trends: (1) increasing asthma prevalence (or frequency) in the American population, (2) increasing trends of death from asthma, and (3) striking differences in hospitalizations, emergency room visits, and deaths from asthma. The disparities were geographic and racial. African Americans in particular continue to have higher rates of asthma-related visits to the emergency department, hospitalizations, and deaths compared to Caucasians.

Additional and more recent statistics from 1980 through 1996 clearly reveal an increase in asthma prevalence in the United States. The data since 1995 show an increase in national rates of office, clinic, and emergency room visits for asthma, in par-

The diagnosis of asthma is too often overlooked, particularly in older age groups and in adolescents, and especially in teenaged girls.

Morbidity

A measure of illness in a given population. The yearly morbidity rate from a disease is defined as the proportion of people affected by that disease per year, per given unit of population.

Mortality

A measure of illness based on the rate of death from a disease in a given community or population at a precise point in time. The yearly mortality rate from a disease is defined as the ratio of deaths caused by that disease to the total number of persons in that community or population.

General Information

allel with a decrease in the rates of hospitalization and death from asthma. Experts believe that the increase in outpatient visits is the result of better asthma treatment combined with increasing rates of asthma. According to the theory, the recorded drop in hospital admissions and deaths from asthma is consistent with improved overall asthma care, which is an encouraging public health statistic.

The reason why asthma is increasing in the United States (and other industrialized countries) is uncertain. Several intertwined causes or factors may be responsible. The topic is certainly a cause of great interest and research, both here and abroad. One theory, called the hygiene hypothesis (see Question 13), concerns childhood asthma and is particularly intriguing. It attempts to explain the increased prevalence of asthma and allergy in affluent, industrialized nations and attempts to discover the factors that may be responsible for the development of asthma.

12. How significant is the problem of asthma in childhood, and what can be done to improve the situation?

Childhood asthma has become a significant problem. More than 20.5 million people have been diagnosed with asthma in the United States; 6.5 million are children younger than 18 years. Of this population, approximately nine hundred thousand are younger than 5 years. The numbers clearly show that despite increasing knowledge and the availability of more effective medications, asthma continues to be a major pediatric health concern. Asthma is without question the most common chronic medical illness affecting children and adolescents in our country.

During the five-year period ending in 1999, almost 14 million days were lost from school each year directly attributable to bronchial asthma. Between 1995 and 1999, asthma accounted for more than 3.5 million medical office visits every year.

Acute asthma was responsible for an average of six hundred thousand emergency room visits for treatment and for almost two hundred thousand hospital admissions each year during the same period. Tragically, between 100 to 200 children die each year from asthma and its complications. What makes the statistic so devastating is the fact that when children receive appropriate medications and ongoing medical care, there should rarely, if ever, be a fatal outcome.

When asthma is accurately diagnosed in children earlier rather than later in the course of the disease, and when self-management education emphasizing the appropriate use of individual medications is provided to both parents and children, asthma statistics in this country will greatly improve. Patient education is the key to opening the door to a new era of enhanced asthma control, which will produce a favorable decline in statistics regarding asthma hospitalization, unscheduled office and emergency room visits, and asthma deaths. The model for achieving better results in the treatment of asthma is the establishment of a true partnership between physician, patient, and parents. When all members of the "team" work together towards the common goal of raising a healthy and active child, the ultimate outcome is a positive one for the entire family, asthma notwithstanding.

Through education, your family will become more knowledgeable about asthma and therefore more comfortable addressing and dealing with the many potentially confusing and occasionally frightening aspects of the disease. For example, if you understand why certain medications are prescribed for your child, you are more likely to follow the dosing recommendations. An important reason why some children may experience difficulty controlling their asthma is that they overuse or, more commonly, under use their medications.

Effective communication and compliance are two crucial components of a successful management program for every asthma patient. Open communication between family and physician is critical to a successful outcome for your child. Medical compliance (or adherence) refers to the consistent daily administration of the medications that have been prescribed for your child. When these two aspects of the management plan are working well, the result is almost always successful and quite gratifying for the patient, parents, and physician.

Frank's comment:

Asthma can be quite significant in childhood, and speaking as one who grew up with the condition, it can be frightening as well. Children seem to be naturally attracted to activities that are extremely physical . . . and often very tiring. When asthma is involved, a simple game of tag can very easily bring on a coughing fit where you are struggling to breathe. Although this can be the same result for adults who engage in similar activities and is scary, to say the least, for a child (especially those who are very young and do not truly understand what asthma is) this can be terrifying. Looking back, I can remember a number of times during my childhood when I suffered from noteworthy asthma attacks. They can very quickly overwhelm a young person, and if the child is not sufficiently prepared, they can be deadly.

13. What is the "hygiene hypothesis"? Is it true that having pets in the house will stop my child from having asthma?

Immune system

The primary defense system of the body, the immune system is responsible for providing protection against bacteria, viruses, cancerous cells, and any proteins that are foreign to the body.

The British epidemiologist David Strachan advanced the hypothesis in 1989 after studying the health records of close to 17,000 British children. The hypothesis proposes that the rising prevalence of asthma and allergic diseases parallels the decreasing prevalence of childhood infections. Over the past century, urbanization, advances in public health (such as immunizations), improved sanitation, and the adoption of cleaner living environments, along with the introduction of antibiotics, have led to reductions in infectious illnesses in children. During the same period, the occurrence of asthma and allergic diseases has increased. The hygiene hypothesis links the two observations. The hypothesis suggests that the reduced exposure to "dirty" environments and infectious agents at a specific point during early childhood leads to stimulation of the part of the growing child's developing immune system that favors the development of allergic conditions, including asthma. Changes consequently fail to occur in the maturing immune response, and the absence of those changes then predisposes that child to an increased risk for developing allergy or asthma.

Epidemiological studies of large groups of people with and without asthma have noted that two environmental factors seem to play a protective role in preventing asthma: attendance at a day care facility before the age of 1 year and the presence of a dog in the family home before birth and onward. Both observations seem to support aspects of the hygiene hypothesis. In the majority of day care facilities, there are almost always children in attendance who have colds; this situation generally leads to a higher incidence of infections among the infants and toddlers in that environment. Additionally, studies have documented a decreased incidence of asthma in children who grew up in rural or farming communities who had close contact with animals early in their lives. The combination of increased numbers of infections, exposure to multiple pets or farm animals, along with fewer immunizations may stimulate the immature immune system to preferentially travel down an immunologic pathway that leads away from allergy and asthma.

Whether there is an age at which a child's immune system must be stimulated in a very specific manner with certain environmental agents, viruses, or bacteria in order to prevent asthma from developing is currently unknown. Dr. Strachan reassessed his hypothesis at the ten-year mark and published a follow-up in the journal *Thorax* in 2000 that summarized other researchers' studies and investigations of the theory. Dr. Strachan concludes that the hypothesis remains "biologically

The hygiene hypothesis proposes that the rising prevalence of asthma and allergic diseases parallels the decreasing prevalence of infections in childhood.

Virus

A type of infectious agent. Viruses contain a single strand of either DNA or RNA, surrounded by a protein coat. Because they only contain one strand of genetic information, viruses cannot replicate on their own and require a host cell for replication. Depending on the particular virus and the underlying health of the human, viral infections can run the gamut from mild to life-threatening.

plausible." The hygiene hypothesis thus remains controversial, and currently represents an interesting, thought-provoking theory that is far from proven. As interesting as these observations may be, asthma specialists require more scientific evidence before accepting the theory. Obviously, no clinical recommendations can be advanced based on the currently available data.

14. No one on either side of our family has asthma, so how could my son develop asthma?

Even though family history and genetic inheritance unquestionably play significant roles in determining if a child will develop asthma, they are not in themselves not "the whole story." In addition to an obvious genetic history in some families with asthma, many other children have the disease without a family history of either allergy or of asthma. In addition to the genetic aspects of asthma, infectious, allergic, and environmental factors play a role in the development of asthma in an individual child. The two major environmental factors associated with the development of asthma are exposure to airborne allergens and viral respiratory infections. Other exposures such as tobacco smoke and air pollutants appear to also be associated with an increased risk for asthma but the relationship is less well defined.

Eczema

An allergic skin condition also known as atopic dermatitis. In babies, eczema often involves the cheeks and the diaper area, whereas in older children a distribution behind the elbow creases and the area behind the knees is classic. Eczema can be very itchy and drying.

Allergic rhinitis

A manifestation of allergy expressed as nasal symptoms with itching, runny nose, and congestion. When caused by seasonal airborne allergens, allergic rhinitis is sometimes referred to as hay fever or rose fever.

The work involved in the search for specific genes responsible for causing asthma in humans is a highly involved and complex process. Within the next decade, geneticists may nonetheless be able to predict through chromosomal analysis who is at risk for the development of asthma and allergy. Recall that a high percentage of children with asthma have associated allergic (most often nasal or skin) conditions. Between 60% and 80% of children with asthma are also allergic. Similarly, approximately 20% of children with allergic rhinitis also have asthma. If your family has no known history of asthma, but there is a positive history of allergic rhinitis (hay fever) or of atopic dermatitis (eczema), then your child also is at an increased risk for developing asthma.

If asthma is not caused solely by a genetic predisposition, what other reasons might explain why a child who has no close relatives with asthma develops this condition? Through decades of clinical observation, physicians have realized that environmental factors play a significant role in the development of pediatric asthma. Viral infections occurring in children younger than five years are probably the most common triggers of asthma-like symptoms in the preschool-aged population. Several classes of viruses seem to be "asthmagenic" which indicates that they have the potential to cause an asthma-like clinical illness. Representatives of these families include the respiratory syncytial virus (RSV), adenoviruses, rhinoviruses, and the influenza virus. After recovery from an illness caused by a strain of one these viruses, susceptible children exhibit increased "irritability" of their lungs. This response pattern is called bronchial hyperreactivity (see Question 8). The heightened level of activity involving the bronchial passageways is a hallmark of asthma. There are many situations, such as another respiratory tract infection, exposure to cold windy weather, or strenuous physical activity, that will cause children with established bronchial hyperreactivity to develop symptoms typical of asthma, such as coughing and wheezing.

Viral infection
An infection caused by or related to a virus.

Influenza
Refers to the influenza virus and the infectious illness caused by that virus in humans. Influenza begins abruptly and is characterized by high fever, chills, aches, and exhaustion. The illness is preventable through vaccination.

Environmental factors associated with changing weather patterns involving extremes of heat or cold, exposure to tobacco smoke, and in some children, emotionally stressful situations are nonallergic precipitants of asthma in nonallergic children. Asthma is a condition that develops not only because of a genetic relationship but also because of allergic, infectious, and environmental factors.

In addition to the genetic aspects of asthma, infectious, allergic, and environmental factors play a role in the development of asthma.

15. Do more boys than girls have asthma?

Yes, but only among children. As young children, boys are almost twice as likely as girls to develop asthma. Interestingly, the pattern seems to be reversed when looking at asthma in older age groups. A study published in the medical journal *Chest* in October 2003 found that 62% of asthma patients younger than

18 years were male, whereas 68% of adult asthma patients were female. Studies of severe asthma in youngsters have also noted a preponderance of boys: two out of three children with severe asthma are boys. However, women account for two-thirds of adults with severe asthma. These gender-based differences are not well understood. Theories suggest the influence of female hormones and the size difference between boys' and girls' lungs as they grow and mature into adulthood.

Hormone

A chemical substance produced in the body by specialized organs called endocrine glands. Once synthesized, hormones circulate in the bloodstream and regulate different body functions.

Kerrin's comment:

I find it interesting that my daughter never suffered from any allergies or asthma, but that my son has been struggling with both since shortly after he was born. After hearing all of the theories as to why this might be, a few pieces seem to fit into the puzzle. Besides the greater tendency for young boys to develop asthma than young girls, my daughter began going to day care in the first year of her life. Of course, when she first started going, she would get sick a lot. Eventually, however, she seemed to adjust to the increased exposure to germs and would only very occasionally get sick. My son didn't start going to day care until after he was 2 years old, and is still very sensitive to germs, often becoming sick on an almost weekly basis, with his asthma symptoms kicking in every time.

16. What are asthma triggers? How can I figure out what triggers my child's asthma?

An asthma trigger is a specific situation or exposure that causes individuals with asthma to develop their typical pattern of asthma symptoms (Table 5). Some triggers, such as exposure to cold air, are considered universal because anyone with asthma who breathes cold air for a long enough time will eventually experience increased symptoms. Those individuals may, for example, notice chest discomfort during the exposure, along with the development of cough and even wheezing. Respiratory infections are another example of an often unavoidable, universal asthma trigger, especially during the winter cold and flu season.

Table 5 Asthma Triggers

Asthma triggers involve situations, conditions, and circumstances that precipitate or worsen a person's asthma. A child with asthma may have more than one trigger. Some triggers are extremely common whereas others are more specific and affect fewer children.

Allergens
  Common examples include pets (cats, dogs, birds), foods (milk, eggs, peanut, tree nuts, shellfish), or aeroallergens (pollen from trees, grasses, weeds, mold spores)

Cold Air

Cigarette Smoke

Exercise

Infections: Viral or Bacterial
  • Bronchitis/Chest colds
  • Pneumonia
  • Sinusitis
  • "Common cold"

Irritants

Medications

Stress

Sulfites

Correctly identifying your child's specific triggers and then avoiding exposure to them, will allow better control of asthma symptoms. Another important treatment strategy involves increasing, or "stepping-up," the dose of asthma medications before an anticipated, unavoidable exposure to a known trigger occurs.

In children younger than 5 years of age, a respiratory tract infection is the most common asthma trigger. Most of these "colds" are caused by viruses. Several classes of viruses seem to be asthmagenic, as discussed in Question 14, meaning that they leave the bronchial passageways in a residual hyperirritable or "twitchy" state following the acute infection. It appears that only children with a predisposition to exhibit asthma symptoms tend to develop bronchial hyperreactivity after an infection with specific viruses. The specific virus families include members of the adenovirus, rhinovirus, respiratory syncytial virus (RSV), and influenza virus families.

In children younger than five years of age, a respiratory tract infection is the most common asthma trigger.

Exercise, especially at high intensity, is also a common asthma trigger. Some children with asthma may only experience asthma symptoms in association with a period of strenuous physical activity. Exercise-induced bronchospasm (EIB), discussed in Question 67, is generally more noticeable with activities that require continuous effort for longer periods. Sports such as soccer, field hockey, lacrosse, cycling, and cross-country running fall into this category. From a seasonal point of view, the fall and winter months are more problematic for children with EIB. Effective medications can control symptoms of EIB; therefore, many doctors do not recommend stopping or modifying a child's athletic activities. They would instead advise medication adjustment and continuation of athletics. Only a very unusual situation would require a doctor today to recommend decreasing a child's level of physical activity.

Other triggers, although far from rare, are specific to individual children and represent examples of allergic sensitization that are unique to a given person and are often referred to as individual triggers. Examples of such triggers include aeroallergens from grass, tree and weed pollen; allergic reactions to foods; and allergens from animals, such as cats, dogs, and mice. Cockroaches and dust mites (see Question 70) are also common triggers. However, outdoor environmental allergens generally do not play a significant role as asthma triggers in children younger than the age of 4 years.

Years ago, asthma was mistakenly believed to be an emotional or psychological condition. Today, physicians understand that this is not the case. However, emotionally stressful situations, which can cause prolonged periods of laughing or crying, can occasionally trigger asthma symptoms. Obviously, neither a physician nor a parent would want to stop a child from laughing or crying, because these are normal, healthy emotional responses; however, it is important to recognize that these emotionally triggered reactions have the potential to precipitate asthma symptoms.

A trigger is best viewed as a medically undesirable stimulus to allergy and asthma. A trigger by definition precipitates the development of allergy symptoms, or of asthma symptoms, or both. A teenager who is allergic to cats will develop itchy eyes and a runny nose after entering a room that contains a cat. His exposure to the cat allergen is the trigger for the emergence of his allergy symptoms, namely the itchy eyes and the runny nose. Similarly, many parents know that their child's asthma symptoms are likely to worsen when they have a viral respiratory infection. In this example, the infection itself is the trigger that stimulates the development of coughing, wheezing, and breathlessness. An essential component of the successful management of a child's asthma is the identification of that child's individual triggers, which should then be avoided as much as realistically possible. If exposure to a specific trigger cannot be avoided (e.g., how does one avoid a cold?), then the treatment strategy shifts from avoidance to proactively increasing your child's medication in consultation with the physician (see Question 32).

Here are possible ways to avoid some of the triggers that may play a role in your child's asthma: during the typical pollen seasons (spring, summer, fall), keep the windows closed, use air conditioners, and avoid having your child in close contact with gardening activities (such as cutting grass or applying chemical fertilizers). Stay away from stores, restaurants, and recreational areas where smoking is permitted. Always inquire whether your child's playmate lives in a house with dogs or cats. These are merely a few examples of some simple actions that can be taken to decrease your child's exposure to potential asthma triggers.

For parents who are careful observers, it may be straightforward to identify factors and situations that are likely to trigger their child's asthma symptoms. Once parents possess this knowledge, the next step is for them to assist their child in avoiding triggers and potentially dangerous situations whenever possible (Table 6). Your child's physician can certainly be a helpful resource; you should not hesitate to mention any trigger you think might be contributing to your child's asthma symptoms.

Table 6   Control of Factors Affecting Asthma Severity

Any of the eight factors described below may contribute to making your child's asthma more difficult to control.

Factor	Control Measure
Allergens	Correctly identify specific allergens and address appropriately with avoidance, antihistamine therapy, or immunotherapy injections. Epinephrine auto-injectors for emergency use might be prescribed.
Tobacco smoke	Smoke-free home and other environments.
Rhinitis	Directed therapy: nasal sprays (cromolyn, nasal steroids), nasal washes, antihistamines, leukotriene antagonists, and decongestants.
Sinusitis	Correct diagnosis is important; drainage measures, washes, nasal steroids, antihistamines and/or decongestants may be prescribed. Antibiotic therapy is reserved for acute bacterial infections.
Gastroesophageal reflux (GERD)	Dietary manipulations, small, frequent feedings, prescription antacid medication. Elevation of the head of the bed may be helpful.
Viral respiratory infections	Yearly influenza vaccination is necessary unless contraindicated (severe egg allergy).
Selected medications*	Beta-blockers in any form; eye drops (used in glaucoma treatment) and pills (used in high blood pressure and heart disease treatment) can cause bronchospasm. Aspirin-sensitive children must avoid aspirin and the nonsteroidal anti-inflammatory class of medicines.
Sensitivity to sulfite additives*	Sulfite-sensitive asthmatics should avoid all sulfite-containing foods. Common examples are dried fruits, and red wine and beer (for adults only, please!).

*These factors are uncommon in children. They are included for completeness as they are important considerations in adult asthma.

General Information

Frank's comment:

An asthma trigger is essentially the finger that knocks down the first domino. From this one action a continuous pattern of reactions can very quickly get out of hand. There are numerous varieties of these "fingers," and each has a different effect on the severity of the result they may cause. Allergies are one kind of trigger (and probably most people's least favorite). Dust, mildew, pollen, and ragweed are my worst enemies. Different diseases and illnesses can also trigger asthma symptoms and attacks. My biggest disappointment growing up was that my extreme love for the winter season brought influenza and colds with it.

Once the domino triggers have been identified, the symptoms and attacks will become more avoidable. One way to do this is to keep careful note of when and where these problems become more frequent. If your child is complaining about feeling "tight" inside his chest ("Mommy, it feels like someone is sitting on me when I breathe.") or is coughing quite a bit every time he or she has been jumping in the autumn leaves, chances are those leaves might be a "finger" trigger. You might consult a respiratory specialist or allergist if just observing isn't cutting it . . . or even just to be on the safe side. Asthma is really all about doing the best you can to prevent those dominoes from falling in the first place. It's going to happen from time to time, but identifying the triggers is a step in the right direction.

Kerrin's comment:

It wasn't difficult to figure out that every time my son got a cold, his asthma symptoms would flare. The doctor gave us our nebulizer the first time our son got a bad cold because he was wheezing. The second time he got a bad cold, he ended up in the hospital for breathing treatments every two hours and had to stay in an oxygen tent. Now whenever he starts to sneeze continually and we see his nose starting to run, we get the nebulizer out and start giving him preventative treatments to try to stave off the worst. We also figured out quickly that another trigger for my son's asthma was exposure to dogs. His second trip to the emergency room, which led to another overnight in the hospital, occurred after visiting my mother's house where two dogs live (even though they are supposed to be "hypoallergenic" dogs, which I was later told by my son's pediatric allergy specialist is impossible no matter what the breed). We haven't been back to my mother's house for well over a year and a half.

17. Does my child need to be allergic to develop asthma?

No. Your child need not be allergic to develop asthma. Similarly, your child's symptom triggers need not be allergic triggers. Asthma triggers can be allergic as well as nonallergic. Studies reveal that high percentage of children with asthma—the majority, in fact—have been found to be allergic; in some studies as high as 70% to 80%. Note that not all asthma is triggered by allergy however. Many children, especially those younger than 5 years, will wheeze only when they have a cold or other infection caused by a virus. Strenuous physical exertion, especially during cold weather, is a common nonallergic trigger that will precipitate symptoms of shortness of breath, chest tightness, cough, or a wheeze. This form of asthma is referred to as exercise-induced bronchospasm or EIB (see Question 67).

Additional nonallergic triggers may involve changing weather patterns, such as cold, windy days or those that are excessively hot and humid. Airborne irritants and pollutants, such as the exhaust from cars and trucks, and indoor exposure to strong odors or cigarette smoke are well-recognized precipitants of asthma. This partial listing of nonallergic triggers for asthma is not intended to be all-inclusive, but merely illustrates the fact that there are many reasons why children who are not allergic can have bronchial asthma. Years ago, asthma was classified as either intrinsic (nonallergic) or extrinsic (allergic). Although the categorization has fallen into disuse, asthma specialists have recognized for many years that one does not have to be allergic to have asthma.

18. What is immunoglobulin E (IgE)?

The immunoglobulins are a family of protein substances whose primary function is to protect the body against infection from bacteria or viruses. Until approximately forty years ago, four members of the immunoglobulin family were recognized: IgG, IgA, IgM, and IgD. The fifth and last member was discovered in 1967 and designated IgE (immunoglobulin E).

IgE has been identified as "the allergic antibody." The protein is considered a marker for the presence of allergic disease. Although an elevation of the total IgE in the blood is not invariably associated with allergy, approximately 60% to 70% of people who have allergic symptoms have an increased total IgE level. A blood test can measure a child's total IgE level as well as specific IgE levels. If a substances such as a specific food, pollen, mold, or animal is suspected of causing a child's asthma and/or allergy symptoms, then a blood test to assay for that specific IgE level should be obtained.

As an example, consider Susan, whose parents got her a beautiful Persian cat for her birthday. Within a week of its arrival, Susan began to experience symptoms consisting of a runny nose, itchy eyes, and nighttime cough. During the next week, her symptoms worsened. Her mother, who had had mild hay fever as a child, became concerned and took Susan to see her doctor. After hearing the history, the doctor became suspicious that Susan might be experiencing an allergic reaction to her new cat. He prescribed an antihistamine and requested that the family call him in five days with a progress report.

After taking the antihistamine, Susan's symptoms decreased, and she felt better, but she was "not 100% back to normal." The doctor then ordered two blood tests: a total IgE level and

Immunoglobulin

A protein produced by the body's immune system as part of an immune response to an antigen.

Immunoglobulin E (IgE)

A type of immunoglobulin that increases and is produced in greater quantity in the setting of atopy, during the course of a typical allergic reaction, and in allergic asthma.

Antibody

A protein molecule produced in blood or tissues in direct response to a foreign substance or antigen. A specific antigen leads to the production of a corresponding specific antibody. Antibody made in response to common environmental agents, such as pollens, grasses, mold, and animal dander, may lead to the development of allergy.

General Information

a specific test for cat IgE. The results showed that Susan had a slightly elevated total IgE and a significantly elevated cat IgE level. Therefore, based on Susan's history and her abnormal IgE levels, the doctor confirmed and documented that her symptoms were caused by an allergy to her newly arrived cat.

Susan's example illustrates a number of points. The first is the need for a detailed history of a child's current symptoms along with a complete present and past family history with special attention to the presence of any family history of allergy. The information Susan's physician obtained made him suspicious that her symptoms were the result of an allergic reaction. Secondly, depending on the severity and duration of a child's symptoms, it would not be inappropriate to see what effect a medication such as an antihistamine would have before proceeding to order laboratory tests. Susan's favorable clinical response to the antihistamine made the doctor more confident of the diagnosis of allergy. Thirdly, in order to confirm his hunch that the cat was the cause of Susan's symptoms, he ordered the IgE measurements. Although the slightly elevated total IgE only suggested that the problem was allergic, the marked increase in the specific cat IgE level proved the doctor's clinical suspicion and documented the diagnosis of cat allergy.

An elevated total IgE level may suggest that a child is allergic, but it is the individual IgE determination for specific allergens (such as pollens, molds, foods, or animals) that confirms that the child is at risk for developing clinical symptoms as a direct result of exposure to a specific allergen.

For several years after the discovery of IgE, some doctors ordered total IgE levels as part of the initial evaluation of new patients. Current thinking is that routinely and automatically measuring every patient's total IgE level is neither clinically helpful nor medically necessary. Elevated total IgE levels can be found in medical conditions other than asthma and allergy.

Persons ill with parasitic infestations or AIDS, for example, as well as active smokers, have elevated blood levels of IgE.

Without question, the discovery and identification of IgE as the allergic antibody has greatly increased the knowledge about the immunologic nature of the allergic reaction. Since then, great strides have been made in understanding the mechanisms underlying conditions such as allergic rhinitis, atopic dermatitis, and allergic asthma.

19. Can asthma permanently damage my child's lungs?

Yes, asthma could cause permanent changes to your child's lungs and yes, modern asthma treatment strives to prevent such damage as much as possible. Asthma specialists believe that the goal of appropriate asthma treatment thus includes control and prevention of asthma symptoms along with normalization of lung function to as great a degree as possible. A major objective of current asthma management is thus the preservation of lung function and the prevention of permanent lung dysfunction.

A pulmonary function test (PFT) is the best way for lung specialists to measure and assess lung function (see Question 37). In particular, the pulmonary function test called spirometry is very useful for following lung function in patients with asthma. Spirometry can be normal in asthma, or it can be abnormal in a particular pattern that is named an "obstructive pattern." The presence of obstructive dysfunction on PFT testing indicates that that person's asthma is not entirely quiescent on that day and at the time that the testing was performed. Spirometry in uncontrolled, symptomatic asthma will reveal increasing obstructive dysfunction. As the asthma is brought under control and symptoms abate, the obstructive dysfunction will also decrease and the values should return to baseline or to normal. A key point about asthma is that it leads to reversible obstructive dysfunction on the spirometry portion of pulmonary function testing. Although there are

Great strides have been made in understanding the mechanisms underlying conditions such as allergic rhinitis and allergic asthma.

Pulmonary function tests (PFTs)

Include the measurement of lung volumes, spirometry, diffusion, and sometimes arterial blood gasses.

Spirometry

A pulmonary function test (PFT) that is the most important PFT in diagnosing and treating asthma. Spirometry measures the flow of air from the lungs as a person forcefully and fully exhales from a deep inspiration. It is used to detect the presence and extent of obstructive dysfunction.

Corticosteroids

Hormones normally produced in very small quantities by the body's adrenal glands that play a role in regulating blood pressure and maintaining the body's salt and water balance. Corticosteroids in inhaled form are a key medication used to treat asthma in all age groups.

several different lung diseases that lead to obstructive dysfunction on testing, only asthma has the potential for reversibility, or normalization, of lung function.

Recall that reversible obstructive dysfunction is usually present to a variable degree when a patient with asthma experiences typical asthma symptoms. As the symptoms lessen and become controlled with medication, the obstructive dysfunction decreases and ideally reverses entirely as lung function normalizes. Poorly controlled asthma will therefore create prolonged periods of obstructive dysfunction, whereas well-controlled asthma will lead to reversal of obstructive dysfunction and normalization (or near-normalization) of lung function, as determined by spirometry. Experts believe that asthma treatment that does not effectively reverse obstructive dysfunction long term may eventually lead to irreversible changes in the air passages, with permanent loss of lung function, or what has been named airway remodeling.

The current view is that: (1) the main abnormality in asthma is inflammation (see Question 8) and (2) long-standing unchecked inflammation is the main culprit in airway remodeling. Asthma experts view asthma as a complex interaction of airflow obstruction, bronchial hyperresponsiveness, and underlying lung inflammation. Children with asthma have a greater inflammation in their lungs and bronchial tubes as compared to children without asthma. Similarly, all children with asthma have increased bronchial hyperreactivity (see Question 8). Bronchial hyperreactivity can be evaluated in a pulmonary function laboratory using a specialized lung test called a methacholine challenge, or bronchoprovocation test (see Question 44).

Medications used to treat bronchial asthma are currently classified into two major groups. In the first group are medications directed toward the relief of early, acute symptoms such as wheezing, coughing, breathlessness, and chest tightness. The short-acting bronchodilator medications are a major example of the fast-acting, quick-relief agents in this group. The second major class of asthma medicines is those prescribed for daily administration to reduce or eliminate inflammation occurring within the bronchial passageways. Examples in this group include inhaled corticosteroids, long-acting broncho-dilators, mast cell stabilizers, and antileukotriene modifiers. Medicines in the first group have been referred to as "rescue" medicines and those in the second as "controllers" in accordance with a terminology proposed by National Asthma Education and Prevention Program (NAEPP) (see Question 48). The 2006 Global Initiative for Asthma (GINA) guidelines for asthma treatment have introduced a revised terminology replacing "rescue" and "controller" with a phraseology that more accurately indicates when the medications should be administered.

Because asthma is a disease of persistent inflammation, and because increased lung inflammation has long-term undesirable effects on lung structure (such as airway remodeling), anti-inflammatory medications, specifically the corticosteroid class of drugs, are the cornerstones of asthma treatment. Inhaled corticosteroid (ICS) formulations have revolutionized the treatment of asthma because they most effectively target underlying lung inflammation. Bronchodilator medicines relieve the wheezing and cough of asthma, but do not treat the inflammation that is the driving force and stimulus to the constriction of the air tubes and the irritation of mucus-producing glands. Inflammation is the major "problem" in asthma and anti-inflammatory medicine is consequently a fundamental part of asthma treatment. The NAEPP, which guided and unified asthma care from 1989 onward, was the first to recommend treating all persistent classifications of asthma (mild, moderate, and severe) with a daily anti-inflammatory medication in addition to bronchodilators. More recent refinements of treatment and classification published by GINA in November and December of 2006 similarly emphasize the use of daily inhaled corticosteroids in controlling childhood asthma. The GINA panel strongly advocates: "Inhaled glucocorticosteroids are the

National Asthma Education and Prevention Program (NAEPP)

A program founded in 1989 under the auspices of the National Institute of Health's National Heart, Lung, and Blood Institute. The NAEPP aims to improve asthma care in the United States by teaching health professionals, asthma patients, and the general public about asthma. The NEAPP's panel of experts has published several expert panel reports with guidelines for the diagnosis and management of asthma.

Global Initiative for Asthma (GINA)

A program launched in 1993 in collaboration with the National Heart, Lung, and Blood Institute, National Institutes of Health, USA, and the World Health Organization. GINA's program is determined and its guidelines for asthma care are shaped by committees made up of leading asthma experts from around the world.

General Information

most effective controller therapy, and are therefore the recommended treatment for asthma for all children of all ages."

Recommended treatment of symptomatic asthma includes anti-inflammatory medication, specifically the inhaled corticosteroid class of drugs.

Physicians specializing in the care of childhood asthma believe that controlling inflammation, minimizing exacerbations, and working toward a symptom-free state make normal or near-normal development of lung function an achievable goal. However, when asthma is inadequately treated and obstructive dysfunction is permitted to continue chronically for long periods, airway remodeling may occur. Airway remodeling refers to subtle changes that affect the structure of the lungs in such a way that the previously reversible component of airway dysfunction characteristic of asthma becomes irreversible. Studies of adults with asthma indicate that once airway remodeling occurs, some degree of lung function is irrevocably lost; it is still unknown whether this is true in children as well. The amount of permanently lost lung function depends on the extent of the airway remodeling change. Current long-term asthma therapy (daily controller therapy) relies heavily on inhaled corticosteroid therapy, rather than on long-term use of oral steroids, to control symptoms and possibly prevent or, in severe cases, at least limit airway remodeling.

20. Is it true that children can actually die from asthma?

Yes. Unfortunately, many people do not understand that asthma can be fatal, even in children. Despite the significant increased understanding of asthma over the past four decades and the improved medications available for treating the condition, the fatality rate has only recently begun to decline. In the United States, approximately four thousand people with a primary diagnosis of asthma die each year. The asthma mortality statistics from the past fifteen years show a slight decrease in the number of deaths in children between the ages of 5 and 18 years. Unfortunately, the exception to this trend has occurred in children younger than age 5. Between 1999 and 2001, the fatality rate increased from 1.7 per million to 2.1 per million in that age group. Most asthma deaths overall occur in adults older than 60 years.

According to statistics from the American Lung Association published in May of 2005, the total number of asthma deaths in the United States has decreased by 8.5% since 1999. However, as encouraging as this statistic may be, any death from asthma is one death too many. The death rate from asthma is highest in African Americans, followed by that in Hispanics, and is lowest in Caucasians. Asthma death rates are significantly higher in the inner-city neighborhoods of most large metropolitan American cities than in suburban or rural areas. Several ongoing large population-based studies are focusing on the reasons for these statistics and on possible approaches to decreasing the fatality rate.

Increased knowledge of asthma and the clinical use of more effective medications should theoretically lead to a decrease in the asthma death rate. Asthma specialists believe that most asthma deaths are preventable tragedies (Table 7). Accordingly, fatal and near-fatal asthma have been the subject of much interest and study by physicians. The more experts can learn about persons who die or almost die of asthma, the better they can plan to prevent additional deaths in the future. Data from the United Kingdom, for example, indicates that childhood asthma deaths there occur in two peak age groups: in preschool children and in teenagers. Additionally, asthma-related deaths in preschool-aged children tend to occur in those children who are hospitalized, whereas teenagers who die of asthma most often experience out-of-hospital deaths. In the latter group, delayed identification of a significant asthma exacerbation and the consequent delayed treatment were major factors contributing to the fatal outcome. In fact, the idea that most asthma deaths are caused by a rapidly progressive form of asthma that worsens dramatically over a very short time, such as a few hours, is a myth. The "lightening bolt, out-of-the-blue" fatal asthma attack is actually a fairly unusual event. Delay in seeking medical care is the most common reason for preventable asthma deaths.

Table 7 Fatal Asthma: Facts

Asthma accounts for about 1 in every 250 deaths worldwide and for more than 4,200 deaths annually in the United States.
Most asthma deaths occur in adults; the death rate among children is decreasing.
Most asthma deaths are preventable and usually reflect underestimation of the severity of an exacerbation along with delay in instituting appropriate medications.
Never ignore new, increasing, or worsening asthma symptoms.
Never delay medical care.

Data from both children and adults with asthma indicate that many who have experienced a life-threatening asthmatic episode may have a reduced ability to sense and identify abnormal respiratory sensations and symptoms such as breathlessness. They are also considered to be at an increased risk for additional episodes or similar attacks of life-threatening asthma in the future. Table 8 lists other factors that play a role in the development of fatal asthma.

Table 8 Fatal Asthma: Some Risk Factors

Prior history of a sudden, rapidly progressive, severe exacerbation.
Prior history of intubation for asthma.
Prior history of treatment in an intensive care unit (ICU) for asthma.
Two or more hospitalizations for asthma in the past 12 months.
Three or more visits to a hospital emergency room (ER) for acute asthma symptoms in the past 12 months.
Either (1) an emergency room visit or (2) a hospitalization for asthma in the last 30 days.
Asthma that requires the use of 2 or more metered-dose inhaler (MDIs) canisters of quick-relief short-acting β_2 agonist medication in the last 30 days.
Severe, uncontrolled symptoms requiring long-term, oral steroid medication, such as prednisone or prednisolone.
Recent steroid taper.

Lack of ability to recognize progressively worsening asthma symptoms.

Asthma occurring in a child who has other chronic conditions such as diabetes or heart disease.

Asthma in a child who lives in socioeconomically disadvantaged circumstances, especially in major urban areas.

Serious superimposed medical illnesses, including psychiatric illness.

The important point about asthma management is to never ignore new respiratory symptoms and to never delay responding to increasing symptoms. Make certain your child tells you if he or she notices any change in breathing, such as uncomfortable or heavy breathing with or without cough, breathlessness, nocturnal awakenings, or wheezing. Help your child follow the asthma action plan and step up the medical regimen. Any time your child experiences increased asthma symptoms, frequent contact with the physician is a critical part of the management plan. Remember that it is always easier to deal with small challenges than to wait until an emergency or a crisis develops. Never, ever ignore your child's complaints of increasing symptoms; they are, after all, feeling uncomfortable and turning to you for help. Often, checking a peak flow level (see Question 37) if your child's physician has prescribed a peak flow monitor will provide important information to assist in the self-management process during a period of increased chest discomfort.

Nocturnal

Taking place or occurring during the nighttime. Asthmatic exacerbations, for example, usually include nocturnal symptoms.

Asthma is a chronic disease that requires that patients take medication regularly for long periods. Patients who do not take their medications as prescribed put themselves at potential risk for experiencing a severe or possibly fatal asthma attack. Compliance or adherence is the term used to indicate that a patient is following the medical regimen outlined by their doctor. When that patient is a young child, it is the parent's responsibility to ensure that the medication is taken consistently and on schedule. It is often difficult for adolescents to understand why they must continue to take their medication even when they feel well and when their asthma is controlled (see Question 64).

In establishing a comprehensive management program, it is critical for the physician to educate the patient and the family about the reasons for using specific medications. Confusion concerning how and why to use medications is one reason why patients become noncompliant. It is extremely important in the overall management of children who have asthma for physicians and parents to establish and maintain effective communication.

It is extremely important in the overall management of children who have asthma for physicians and parents to establish and maintain effective communication.

21. I have heard that some children may outgrow their asthma. Is it possible to determine whether my child will be one of those children?

Many pediatricians erroneously equate the disappearance of asthma symptoms over time with what they term "outgrowing" asthma, as discussed further in Question 22. There is no way to know in advance if any particular child will stop experiencing asthma symptoms. Certain historical facts and clinical clues may however provide your physician with enough information for him to hazard an educated guess as to the likelihood of symptoms lessening over time.

The absence of a parental history of allergy on both sides of the family is very favorable prognostic information. A child whose mother currently has (or previously had) asthma, on the other hand, is more likely to have lasting asthma symptoms. If a young child only wheezes when he or she has a cold, the potential for the asthma to disappear increases. The age at first symptom onset is important too, as developing asthma later in childhood makes it more likely that the condition will persist over time. In other words, the older children diagnosed with asthma are when they begin to wheeze, the less of a chance that their symptoms will spontaneously disappear with the passage of time. Ongoing asthma has been associated with the presence of: (1) clinical symptoms of both asthma and eczema, (2) wheezing that develops in the absence of infection, and

(3) physician-diagnosed allergic rhinitis in a child who has experienced previous episodes of asthma.

Many children who have asthma during their early childhood years become symptom-free as adolescents. The observation has prompted some physicians who care for children with asthma to state that a child has outgrown his asthma. Unfortunately, the 24-year-old who begins to wheeze again for the first time since he was 14 years old generally does not call his former pediatrician to report this medical development. Asthma is truly a chronic disease for most individuals. Many children with asthma will, however, also experience long periods without active chest symptoms, a well-known phenomenon that asthma specialist refer to as a state of "prolonged asthma remission." Despite the fact that prolonged asthma remissions occur and may last many years, physicians should never promise any parent that a child will outgrow his or her asthma.

22. Can asthma be cured?

The answer depends what is meant by the word "cured." Asthma is a lifelong condition and therefore can never be truly cured. The state of baseline hyperreactivity (discussed in Question 8) that defines asthma never disappears. At the same time, remember that asthma is a disease with tremendous variability. In many children, especially those with easily controlled asthma, symptoms can remain inactive for long periods. Doctors have also noted that asthma may become less symptomatic and easier to control in many children as they grow through adolescence. In other words, asthma symptoms and the requirement for medication in some children with mild asthma seem to disappear during adolescence.

Many well-intentioned pediatricians, despite evidence to the contrary, still inform parents that a child will grow out of their asthma over time. However, the facts speak otherwise. A child with physician-diagnosed asthma is viewed as having

General Information

Pediatrician
A medical specialist who has received intensive training in the care and treatment of children from birth to young adulthood.

a lifelong condition. It has been recognized that a significant proportion of children with asthma become asymptomatic as they reach adolescence. The absence of chest symptoms for years can understandably lead a pediatrician to conclude that their adolescent patient's asthma has disappeared. Because pediatricians rarely care for their patients after they reach their late teens or early twenties, they will be unaware that their former patient's asthma symptoms have returned. Typically, adults in their late twenties or thirties who develop asthmatic symptoms will recall having had mild asthma as a child and are surprised that they continue to have asthma in adulthood or, as they describe, have it "come back after so many years." Contemporary medical thinking views the phenomenon of disappearing asthma as a state of prolonged asthma remission.

Why, then, would any pediatrician tell a parent that their child's asthma is likely to disappear when they become adults? Are they just trying to be reassuring? You must remember that pediatricians are speaking from the perspective of a physician who only treats children; their patients are not adults. Typically, a pediatrician cares for children until they are between 18 and 21 years of age, a time when asthma can become dormant but not truly cured.

It is virtually impossible to make accurate predictions about the future natural history of one individual child's asthma. We are primarily concerned with treating the current condition, the "here and now," and we focus our energies on achieving a symptom-free state for your child as rapidly as possible. Childhood asthma must be taken seriously and treated correctly to ensure the best possible outcome for your child. Good control of asthma symptoms permits your child to enjoy a full life with time for school, leisure activities, and sports. If this approach provides your child with a long symptom-free period without the need for medication, all the better.

23. My son wheezes and coughs; should I bring him to a specialist? Should he see a lung specialist (a pulmonologist) or an allergy specialist (an allergist)? How many visits will it take the doctor to tell me if my son has asthma?

As a general guideline, a child who has had two or more acute wheezing episodes would benefit from consultation with either a pediatric pulmonologist or an allergist, or even possibly both. Most children with symptoms of recurring cough or wheeze can be fully evaluated for the possibility of asthma within two or three office or clinic visits. It would be an unusual situation for the workup to take any longer. Your child's primary care doctor will most likely be the one to recommend that you bring your child to see a specialist. The decision regarding the timing of the specialty consultation depends on whether the consultation is for evaluation of new symptoms in a child without known asthma, or whether the consultation seeks to improve on existing asthma therapy and management. Answers to questions concerning the frequency and severity of your child's chest symptoms, his response to medication, the presence or absence of nighttime symptoms, and the overall effect that the condition has on his quality of life will help determine if and when a consultation with an asthma specialist is necessary. A child whose asthma is uncontrolled will also benefit from consultation with a physician who specializes in the diagnosis and treatment of childhood asthma.

From a specialist's point of view, asthma can be well managed by either an allergist or a pulmonologist. Does it make a difference which doctor you see? Is there a specific reason why you should have a consultation with one specialist and not the other? Physicians who specialize in allergy or pulmonology will provide excellent care and management of your child's asthma, but you must understand where their expertise overlaps and how it differs.

Pulmonologist

A physician specialist with extra training and qualifications in the diagnosis and treatment of lung diseases.

General Information

47

The major factor to consider when deciding which type of asthma specialist should evaluate your child relates to the role that allergy may have in causing your child's asthma. Data from various studies indicates that between 60% to 80% of children who have bronchial asthma also have allergies. If a child has a family history of allergy or asthma, and particularly if the mother has asthma, there is a strong probability that the child will also develop the condition. Pulmonologists are trained to diagnose and treat diseases of the lungs and are knowledgeable about allergy as it relates to asthma. Allergists, on the other hand, have undergone in-depth training in clinical allergy, are qualified to administer immunotherapy, and diagnose and treat all different types of allergy—including allergy that often accompanies asthma in children. Since asthma in most children tends to be a lung disease with a strong allergic component, it "overlaps" the specialties of both the pulmonologist and of the allergist.

A board-certified allergist has had extensive training in and clinical experience with both asthma and allergy. If you exclude patients with nasal allergy problems, most pediatric allergists spend the majority of their practice time caring for children with bronchial asthma. If there is a suspicion that allergy is playing a significant role in your child's asthma, and especially if your child is thought to be a candidate for "allergy shots" (immunotherapy), then specialty consultation should definitely include an allergist.

Before the age of two or three, most children with asthma do not have a significant allergic component to their disease. In a high percentage of older children and adolescents with asthma, however, allergy plays an important underlying role. Depending on your child's history and particular asthma manifestations (including his or her symptom triggers), a thorough allergy evaluation may well be an important component of a comprehensive asthma evaluation. If your child is initially seen by a pediatric pulmonologist, it may be necessary for him to be seen by an allergist as well at some point in order to complete the diagnostic workup.

We strongly belive that if your child's asthma symptoms are not controlled, if your child has been hospitalized with a severe asthma episode, or if your child has also been diagnosed with a second, complicating condition (such as sinus infections or allergic rhinitis), your child should be seen in consultation by an asthma specialist. Finally, remember that if you, the parent of a child with asthma, are not satisfied with your child's progress or if you believe that there is room for improvement in asthma control, it is entirely appropriate to seek a consultation with a specialist as well. Indications for specialty referral are presented in Table 9.

Table 9   Specialist Referral
Referral to a pediatric asthma specialist is recomended for:

Diagnosis:
- For specialized evaluation including: allergy testing, pulmonary function tests, broncoprovocation test
- If unusual or atypical signs or symptoms are present.

Treatment:
- To regulate and monitor the ongoing adminstration of inhaled corticosteroids in children and adolescents with chronic asthma symptoms
- If it has not been possible to achieve and maintain control of your child's asthma
- For the purpose of educating the child, parents, and caregivers about asthma
- To teach appropriate asthma self-management skills and techniques to both parent and child
- For allergy immunotherapy.

Severity:
- For any child who has been hospitalized for asthma within the past 12 months
- For the child who required oral steriods (burst dosing) three times in a year.

Sinus

Air-filled cavities within the human skull. Adults have several sinuses, named by location: the frontal, ethmoid, sphenoid, and maxillary sinuses. The sinuses continue to form after birth; consequently, the frontal and sphenoid sinuses are not well developed in children.

General Information

49

PART TWO

History, Symptoms, and Physical Examination

Do all children with asthma have similar symptoms?

What exactly is a wheeze?

What are asthma attacks and exacerbations and why are both terms used?

More . . .

24. Do all children with asthma have similar symptoms?

The classic, although not most common, symptom of childhood asthma is intermittent wheezing. A wheeze is an abnormal whistling sound typically heard as a child breathes out, or exhales. Many young children, particularly those younger than 5 years, may instead present with coughing as their only asthma symptom. Cough is the single most common symptom of childhood asthma. Some children may complain of uncomfortable chest tightness or an almost painful heaviness. Children with asthma may experience shortness of breath with exertion, although it can be difficult for them to put that sensation into words and communicate it to others. Although all children with asthma do not exhibit the same pattern of symptoms, most of them have a combination of symptoms that may include wheezing, coughing, chest tightness, and/or breathlessness (Figure 3).

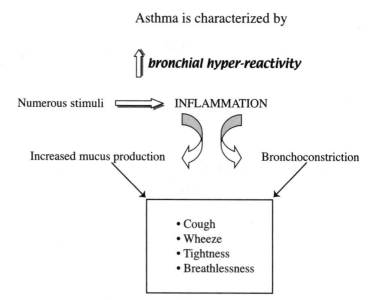

Figure 3   Asthma characteristics.

From a diagnostic perspective, asthma presents with a limited range of clinical symptoms. Lung conditions other than asthma can, however, present with manifestations similar to those of asthma, with coughing and wheezing for instance. The differential diagnosis of asthma and the evaluation of children with symptoms such as coughing, wheezing, chest pain, and breathlessness may on occasion become complex. Nonetheless, most children who have asthma usually exhibit an easily recognized pattern of symptoms.

Most children who have asthma usually exhibit an easily recognized pattern of symptoms.

25. What exactly is a wheeze?

A complete physical examination includes listening to the lungs (auscultation) with a stethoscope. The physician places the chest piece of the stethoscope on the child's chest and upper back and listens as air enters and exits the lungs. The patient (if old enough to comply) is then asked to take several deep breaths, breathing through his or her mouth. The physician pays close attention to any differences in the breath sounds comparing the right and left lungs as well as to any audible abnormalities. The in-and-out movement of air through the lungs and tracheobronchial tree should always be smooth. A wheeze is an abnormal sound produced by turbulent flow of air through the lungs' breathing tubes.

A wheeze refers to an abnormal breath sound made when air travels though a breathing passage (airway) that has become narrowed. The narrowing can be caused by mucus secretions trapped in the airway or by the airway muscles' excessive constriction or tightening. In asthma, airway narrowing is reversible. Bronchodilator medications rapidly help the narrowed airway return to its normal size. A wheeze is best described as a high-pitched whistling sound. Wheezing can occur while breathing in (inspiratory wheezing, occurring during the inspiratory phase of the breath), while breathing out (expiratory wheezing, occurring during the expiratory phase of the breath), or during the entire breathing cycle. Asthma is one of several conditions that can cause wheezing. If wheezing is severe, it can be heard without a stethoscope.

Auscultation

The process of listening to the sounds of air moving in and out of the breathing passages. Auscultation is performed by the examiner placing their stethoscope on the skin overlying the chest and having the patient breathe in and out.

Stethoscope

A medical instrument used to amplify and listen to sounds produced by internal organs, such as the lungs, hearts, or bowels, during a physical examination.

Inspiratory

Refers to breathing in.

Expiratory

Refers to breathing out.

53

Wheezing in asthma reflects ongoing lung inflammation and airway narrowing, or bronchoconstriction. The presence of wheezing indicates that the asthma is active and inadequately controlled and that more intensive stepped-up treatment is necessary (Table 10). Wheezing is never normal and should never be ignored. When airway narrowing and inflammation remain untreated, there is a real risk of worsening of the disease, which can become potentially life-threatening.

Table 10   Asthma: Inactive versus Active

Silent Asthma Inactive / Controlled	Noisy Asthma Active / Not Controlled
Quiescent, asymptomatic asthma No cough or wheeze	Symptomatic, exacerbated asthma with coughing and wheezing
Inflammation absent	Increased, ongoing, active inflammation
Air passages are clear of mucus	Mucus production increases —leads to cough
Air tubes (bronchial passages) are patent, "fully" open	Air tubes narrowed, constricted —leads to wheezing, cough, tightness

26. My 8-year-old son sometimes makes a kind of whistling sound when he breathes. Does that mean that he has wheezing and asthma?

Asthma is a very likely cause of your son's intermittent and recurrent noisy breathing, although your pediatrician will need more details and information to confidently diagnose the cause. Repeated bouts of wheezing in school-aged children—boys and girls—are almost always caused by asthma. The likelihood of asthma is even greater when a cough accompanies wheezing. A family history of asthma or allergy, as discussed in Question 5, is an important risk factor for the development of asthma. Not all children who wheeze however have asthma. Medical evaluation of a child who is wheezing must rule out other possible causes for the wheeze in order to establish the diagnosis (Table 11). The list of such possibilities is called the differential diagnosis. Causes of wheezing in children include congenital abnormalities, such as tracheal webs; various types of infections; tumors; cardiac conditions; and other illnesses, such as cystic fibrosis.

Table 11   Causes of Wheezing in Children

Wheezing is a major asthma symptom; children with recurring episodes of wheezing likely have asthma. Not all children who wheeze, however, have asthma.

Conditions other than asthma that can cause wheezing in children include:

Anatomic abnormalities
 • Bronchopulmonary dysplasia
 • Hypertrophy of tonsils and/or adenoids
 • Primary ciliary dyskinesia
 • Retrognathia (Pierre-Robin syndrome)
 • Tracheal stenosis
 • Tracheo-bronchomalacia
 • Vascular rings

Cardiomegaly

Cystic fibrosis

Foreign body aspiration

Gastroesophageal reflux

Infections of the lung, epiglottis, tonsillar area
 • Bronchiolitis
 • Bronchitis
 • Epiglottitis
 • Peritonsillar abscess
 • Retropharyngeal abscess
 • Tracheitis (bacterial)

Tumors

Vocal cord dysfunction (VCD)

An important cause of nonasthma wheezing, particularly in young children, is called foreign body aspiration. Toddlers (and even older children, much to their parents' dismay) who cannot resist putting small objects in their mouths can occasionally aspirate those foreign bodies, which can then become lodged in the lungs. Similarly, food can be swallowed "down the wrong tube," especially when a child is talking and chewing simultaneously. If it is not immediately coughed up and expelled, the food particle can become firmly lodged in a bronchial passageway. Any aspirated foreign body can cause wheezing and will always require removal of the object from the bronchial passageways. In 2000, foreign body aspiration was reportedly responsible for more than seventeen hundred emergency room visits by children younger than 14 years. Specialists estimate that 80% of foreign body aspirations occur in children younger than 3 years, with peak incidence between 1 and 2 years of age, and more often involve boys.

Incidence

In medicine, refers to the number of new cases of a disease at any point in time.

Medical journals have reported that all types of objects have been retrieved from children's respiratory passages: coins, marbles, pits, and small toys are all on the list. In the United States, peanuts account for up to half of all aspirated foreign bodies in children. Infants and toddlers tend to aspirate food items, whereas older children tend to aspirate nonfood items. It is a wise precaution to cut grapes into quarters before serving them to your 2-year-old. Similarly, if hot dogs or sausages must be on your toddler's menu, do not present them in a bun. Instead, make sure you cut the meat lengthwise and then into smaller pieces before serving. Interestingly, studies have shown that uninflated toy balloons are the objects most commonly implicated in fatal childhood foreign body aspiration, along with spherical toys such as marbles and small balls.

Bronchitis

An inflammation of the lining of the larger bronchial tubes. Bronchitis can be acute, such as from infection, or chronic, such as in the case of tobacco abuse.

Asthma is often underdiagnosed or missed in children. As any parent knows, children frequently catch many colds each year, especially when school is in session. Some children with undiagnosed asthma are erroneously thought to have recurrent chest infections when they in fact have asthma. It is important for specialists to distinguish asthma from repeated episodes of bronchitis and infections, such as pneumonia. Do not assume that your child is experiencing a bad winter if he seems to be getting chest cold after chest cold; he may have asthma (Table 12). If so, make sure your child gets appropriate medical care to establish an accurate diagnosis and receive correct treatment.

Table 12 Is the Diagnosis Asthma?

The ability to accurately establish a diagnosis of asthma in a child is enhanced when certain symptoms are present. The diagnosis may be less straightforward in child with atypical symptoms.

Here are some important symptoms to report and review with your child's doctor:
- The presence of wheezing
  including any pattern of presentation and the identification of any particular obvious precipitating causes.
- The presence of cough and its nature (such as wet, dry, and/or productive) and the situations that seem to cause this symptom, such as exposure to certain environments (for example: near pets, when in a smoke filled restaurant, or around strong perfumes) at certain seasons of the year (for example: in the spring).
- Abnormal and/or uncomfortable sensations of breathing or, in medical terms, *dyspnea*.
- Occurrence of episodic chest tightness or pressure.
- Decrease in exercise tolerance, which limits participation in exercise or sports.
- Nighttime chest symptoms such as cough, wheeze, and/or chest tightness that awaken your child from sleep.
- Lingering "colds" that "always go to the chest" and last more than 10 days or so.

In addition to analyzing the patient's symptoms, the physician will rely on additional data:
- Past medical and family history: any personal or family history of asthma, allergy, or conditions such as eczema or hay fever.
- Results of specialized testing such as:
  Pulmonary function tests (PFTs)
  Peak expiratory flow (PEF) monitoring
  Chest X-rays (may occasionally be required)
  Allergy testing, either directly (prick/puncture or intradermal skin testing) or indirectly (by a blood [RAST®/ImmunoCAP®] test).

27. Our son frequently awakens at around 2:00 a.m., coughing. His doctor previously prescribed an inhaler to be used in case of wheezing. Will the inhaler help treat the cough too? Is it a good idea to have him use his inhaler and let him go back to sleep?

If your son awakens in the early morning with coughing, wheezing, or uncomfortable breathing, he is experiencing what asthma specialists refer to as nocturnal awakenings, which are nocturnal asthma symptoms. Nocturnal awakenings caused by asthma are not normal and are undesirable from many perspectives. Apart from interfering with sleep and rest, they indicate that your child's asthma is not adequately controlled and that it is worsening. Nocturnal awakenings should always be reported to the treating physician. In the National Asthma Education and Prevention Program (NAEPP) classification, an older child with intermittent asthma experiences no more than two nocturnal awakenings in a month. If a child experiences three or more episodes of nocturnal awakenings or chest symptoms in a month, their asthma becomes classified as persistent. Children with moderate persistent and severe persistent asthma by definition, experience weekly nocturnal awakenings. In the updated 2006 Global Initiative for Asthma (GINA) classification, any nocturnal asthma awakenings or nighttime symptoms lead to an asthma classification of "Partly Controlled" at best, and if additional features were present, to a classification of "Uncontrolled" asthma.

When your child awakens with asthma symptoms, it is a good idea for him to use his quick-relief, short-acting, inhaled bronchodilator. It usually is effective; his asthma symptoms should respond and resolve quickly, allowing him (and you) to go back to sleep. When your son awakens in the morning, you need to give some thought to the nighttime episode. If his asthma was previously under good control, try to figure out why he developed nocturnal symptoms. Did he omit (or simply forget) his daily asthma medicine? What was his last peak expiratory flow (PEF) measurement (see Question 37)? Was he exposed to any known triggers? Could he be developing a viral infection?

If your child has experienced two or more nighttime asthma episodes ("awakenings") in the past thirty days, his current medication regimen should be reviewed with the treating physician to ensure compliance and decide if any medication or lifestyle changes are necessary. Remember, with a disturbed sleep pattern, no one can function normally.

28. My 16-year-old daughter thinks that her asthma worsens each month related to when she gets her period. Is that possible?

Thirty to forty percent of women with asthma who menstruate experience exacerbations of their asthma symptoms associated with their menstrual cycle. They consistently note increased asthma symptoms just before and during their period. This phenomenon has been termed premenstrual asthma. Hormonal changes, possibly related to rises in leukotriene levels, have been studied as a possible explanation for the increase in asthma symptoms. The first step in treating premenstrual asthma is to identify whether it is, in fact, present. A symptom diary together with daily peak flow recordings can be helpful. If confirmed, premenstrual asthma can be treated with one or more of the following, depending on symptom severity and individual characteristics: (1) stepped-up anti-inflammatory controller medicine, (2) a trial of oral leukotriene modifiers, and (3) in severe cases, hormone therapy or oral contraceptive medication to suppress ovulation.

Peak Expiratory Flow (PEF)

The PEF is part of the several different measurements obtained during the spirometry portion of PFTs. Because exacerbations of asthma lead to decreasing values of PEF, self-monitoring at home of PEF in asthma is part of contemporary asthma management.

Leukotriene

Inflammatory molecules of which one family in particular, called the cysteinyl-leukotriene, is important in asthma and allergy. Cysteinyl-leukotrienes are released in increased numbers during asthma exacerbations.

29. Are there any unusual physical findings (characteristics) that may indicate that a child either has asthma or is likely to develop bronchial asthma?

This question is easy to answer: no abnormal physical findings are present in children who currently have or may at some future time develop bronchial asthma. You cannot tell if a child has asthma or is likely to develop the condition simply by looking for an abnormality on physical exam. During active asthma, however (termed "partly controlled" and "uncontrolled" in the GINA classification), typical symptoms such as cough or wheeze caused by bronchospasm are usually present. Other signs may include more rapid rate of breathing. During a particularly severe episode, or "asthma attack," breathing is visibly labored, and a child's chest may take on a rounded appearance, known as a barrel chest. The unusual configuration develops as air becomes trapped in the lungs and is exhaled through constricted and inflamed bronchi.

Although it isn't truly a physical finding associated with asthma, there is a definite link between the presence of eczema early in childhood, which is easily detected on visual inspection of the skin, and the subsequent development of asthma. A positive family history of asthma coupled with findings of eczema in a young child indicates a strong probability that the child will exhibit asthma symptoms by the age of five. This pattern of response is consistent with the concept known as the "allergic march" (see Question 31).

No anatomic changes can make pediatricians suspect that asthma is present. Asthma is diagnosed based on a child's history, the physical findings during periods of active symptoms, and the clinical response to bronchodilator and anti-inflammatory medications.

30. I have heard that asthma is primarily a psychological disease. What do experts believe?

Asthma is definitely not a psychological disease; it is a physical condition that affects the lungs and bronchial passages. The concept that asthma is somehow an emotional disturbance is a myth. A child (or adult) who is having difficulty breathing with cough, increased chest pressure, and wheezing is physically extremely uncomfortable. The physical discomfort, coupled with an inability to breathe normally, adds up to an extremely frightening experience. Until normal, unlabored, and comfortable breathing is reestablished, any person in the midst of an asthma attack feels as if they are suffocating. It should come as no surprise that emotions of fear and even panic occur under these circumstances. These misinterpreted emotional responses are a consequence of the asthma attack and not the cause of the episode.

A second reason why asthma might erroneously be considered a psychological condition is the observation that some persons with known asthma develop active symptoms after experiencing very strong emotion, such as shock or grief. The appropriate strong emotional response acts a trigger for asthma symptoms rather than as an underlying cause of the disease itself.

The concept that asthma is somehow an emotional disturbance is a myth.

Emotional upset can sometimes bring on physical symptoms. A child (or adult) may, for example, experience a belly ache in response to an unpleasant or stressful situation. Similarly, some children's asthma symptoms may worsen when they confront a situation they experience as stressful. Whether it is related to school, family members, or other children, it is important that parents, caregivers, and teachers recognize the potential association between asthma symptoms and such harmful stress. Developing working strategies to effectively manage a child's psychological stress, if present, should include your child's physician and is a component of comprehensive asthma care.

31. What are the most common allergens and allergic conditions that affect infants, children, and adolescents?

The term "allergy" as commonly used refers to reactions caused by specific allergens, such as food, dust mites, pollen, and animal dander. "Allergic conditions" is a good term to describe specific clinical illnesses, such as allergic asthma or eczema. Infants possess the immunologic capability to become allergic, and allergic reactions to food in particular occur early in a child's life. The foods that most frequently trigger allergic reactions in infants and young children are milk, eggs, soy, and wheat. Other foods responsible for reactions in the pediatric population include peanut, tree nuts, fish, and shellfish. Of course, many of these foods are not consumed by infants, but are commonly introduced into the diet as a child grows older. A nursing infant, however, is exposed through breast milk to all of the foods the mother eats.

Allergic reactions to food can be observed early in a child's life.

Some children with food allergies develop eczema, or atopic dermatitis. Eczema typically occurs during infancy and can vary widely in its severity. For some children, it is a mild annoyance, but for others it is a major problem. The good news concerning eczema is that most children with this condition do outgrow their symptoms sometime between the ages of 4 and 7. Less often, nasal congestion and/or a runny nose can occur from an allergic reaction to a food. For example, one 2-week-old girl developed severe breathing difficulties because of an allergic reaction to her cow's milk–based infant formula. She developed marked swelling of the membranes in her nose, which caused her to have respiratory distress every time she tried to drink her formula. When the milk-based formula was changed to an infant soy formula, the infant's allergic reaction disappeared and her symptoms resolved. Asthma symptoms consisting of cough or wheeze can thus develop during a child's first year of life, most often triggered by a viral infection or possibly an allergic reaction to a food.

As children who have a genetic predisposition to develop allergies mature from infancy to toddlerhood to preschool age, there is an increasing incidence of allergy symptoms involving the upper and lower airways. It takes years for a potentially allergic child to become sensitized to airborne and environmental allergens. In the home, cats, dogs, dust mites, and cockroaches are the most commonly found allergens. Most outdoor allergens consist primarily of pollen from trees, grasses, and weeds, as well as spores produced by molds. Reactions to these allergens can cause allergic rhinitis (rose or hay fever) with typical symptoms of sneeze, runny nose, and congestion, and the cough and wheeze associated with bronchial asthma. A child who has both eczema and seasonal allergic rhinitis may occasionally experience a flare-up of skin symptoms during the peak of the pollen season.

As children grow older, many who were allergic to foods as infants and toddlers lose those sensitivities. However, reactions to certain highly allergenic foods such as peanut, tree nuts, fish, and shellfish may never disappear and can be lifelong.

Although there are exceptions, it appears that many children exhibit a continuum of allergic symptoms that initially affect the skin (eczema), progress to the nose (rhinitis), and finally involve the lungs (asthma). Researchers are currently investigating possible methods of slowing down or stopping what has been referred to as the allergic march. The hope is that, in the not-too-distant future, through medical research, physician–scientists will develop techniques and procedures that will effectively control and ultimately cure allergic diseases.

Kerrin's comment:

My son developed eczema as an infant. It was particularly bad on his face, and he would develop patches that would not heal no matter what we treated them with, until we finally had to use a steroid cream. He would also occasionally develop hives after breastfeeding, and at 6 months I finally had to wean him because I was down to eating almost nothing for fear that I would induce an allergic reaction, because we could never quite pinpoint exactly what he was allergic to. His eczema eventually went away, but it was replaced with asthma. I was told that this is not unusual, for young children with eczema to later develop asthma.

32. What does my doctor mean by an exacerbation of asthma? Why are the terms attacks *and* exacerbations *both used?*

Pulmonary symptomatology

Symptoms related to the lungs and the act of breathing. Wheezing, coughing, breathlessness, and mucus production are examples of pulmonary symptomatology.

Dyspnea

An abnormal awareness of breathing; a kind of breathlessness.

The first point is that your doctor sounds like a physician who is either an asthma specialist or a doctor who is knowledgeable on the subject. Asthma is characterized by periods of exacerbation and remission. An exacerbation of asthma refers to an increase in lung inflammation and represents a period of increased asthma activity. It indicates a flare of the disease. An exacerbation of asthma is manifested as the development of pulmonary symptomatology. Simply put, this means that your child is actively experiencing increased levels of typical asthma symptoms such as wheezing, coughing, nighttime symptoms, increased mucus production from the lungs, breathlessness or dyspnea, and chest pressure, tightness, or discomfort (Table 13).

Table 13   Asthma Exacerbations: Symptoms

Symptoms are what an individual experiences. Physicians should always ask patients with asthma to report their symptoms.

Dyspnea, an abnormal awareness of breathing
"I feel my breathing; my breathing is uncomfortable."

Breathlessness, at first with exertion or activity; may also occur at rest as an exacerbation progresses
"I can't catch my breath; I'm out of breath and need air."

Cough
"I have an annoying cough; am I sick?"

Mucus production, usually not discolored
"I'm bringing up some clear stuff."

Nocturnal awakenings, interrupted sleep from difficulty breathing
"I keep waking up at 2 a.m. and have problems breathing."

Pressure sensation over chest, or feelings of mid-chest tightness
"I feel as if there's an elephant sitting on my chest."

Wheezing
"It feels like a noise in my chest; my breathing makes a whistling sound."

During an exacerbation, measurement of peak flow and other lung function values will usually decrease. Measurement of lung function also typically reflects reduced values. An exacerbation usually begins with mild symptoms. If unchecked, a mild exacerbation will worsen and become more severe. Mild exacerbations that are identified early and treated appropriately, perhaps through increased use of inhaled medication, can be controlled with minimal, if any, disruption of health and lifestyle. More advanced exacerbations may, however, require additional medications, such as an oral steroid available in tablet or liquid form. Severe or rapidly progressive exacerbations require hospital-based or emergency department intervention and treatment.

Note that the term asthma "exacerbation" has supplanted the outdated concept of asthma "attack" in the medical scientific literature. Exacerbation more accurately describes the gradual nature of the build-up in lung inflammation during disease flares. Many practicing pediatricians and pediatric asthma and allergy specialists (along with the media) prefer to use the term asthma attack in speaking with their patients, especially younger children. Others, especially asthma specialists caring for adults rather than children, believe that the word "attack" implies unpredictability, violence, and vulnerability, whereas the more neutral and descriptive term, "exacerbation," emphasizes potential transience and reversibility. No matter which terminology you and your child's physician use when speaking, an exacerbation of asthma, even of the milder type, should never be ignored or dismissed as insignificant (Table 14).

Treatment of an asthma exacerbation includes a search for factors responsible for loss of asthma control. Did the wheezing recur because of a respiratory infection? Were the several missed doses of medication the culprit? Could the class trip to the petting zoo have been a contributing factor? Correct identification of asthma triggers (see Question 16) not only allows for a better understanding of a child's asthma but also leads to a more proactive approach to asthma management with an emphasis on preventive measures. Learning to increase asthma medicines when certain infectious symptoms develop, for instance, can help prevent a flare or exacerbation. Another example of proactive asthma treatment might include increasing the dose of your child's antiallergy medication before a trip to the zoo if animals are asthma triggers. The stepped-up treatment might be effective in preventing and avoiding asthma symptoms from developing.

Learning to increase asthma medicines when certain symptoms develop can help prevent a flare or exacerbation.

Table 14   Asthma Exacerbations: Key Points

An exacerbation of asthma reflects increased lung inflammation. An exacerbation is a flare of disease activity sometimes referred to as an asthma "attack."

Quick and appropriate intervention and response to increasing symptoms will limit their duration and speed up return to normal lung function. Most exacerbations will require the administration of a "burst" of oral corticosteroid medication.

Although asthma exacerbations develop and generally build gradually, symptoms can rapidly worsen and may lead to hospitalization, respiratory failure, and even death if untreated.

Never ignore increasing or worsening symptoms such as wheezing, cough, nighttime awakenings, or chest tightness. Not all symptoms need to be present in order to have an exacerbation.

Lung function measurements (such as the peak flow, the FEV_1, and the FVC/FEV_1 ratio) usually decrease during an exacerbation.

A major goal of current asthma management includes prevention of exacerbations.

Remember that asthma is a controllable condition with proper treatment.

PART THREE

Diagnostic Evaluation and Workup

How can I find out if my child has allergies?

How does a doctor diagnose asthma?

How will I know if my son's asthma attack is severe enough to require a trip to the emergency room?

More . . .

33. How can I find out if my child has allergies?

Many parents wonder if their child might be allergic to a specific food or an aeroallergen, such as pollen or cat dander. A keen parental observer might notice that after exposure to a cat, for example, their child consistently develops a pattern of symptoms such as itching, redness, and tearing of the eyes. Another child, however, might exhibit less obvious allergic symptoms and a parent might not immediately make the connection. In yet another scenario, the primary care physician will be the one to suspect that a child's recurring pattern of symptoms is related to allergy rather than to another process such as an infection. Either way, consultation with an allergist can be extremely productive and is highly recommended to either confirm or rule out once and for all the diagnosis of allergy.

Allergists are experts in evaluating and caring for children and adults who have allergic diseases. Evaluation always begins with a highly detailed history of the patient's symptoms. Additional information about the child's health and that of his or her parents is also part of a comprehensive allergy evaluation. The physical examination places particular emphasis on the skin, upper respiratory tract, and lungs. Important clues to diagnosing allergy often are found on close inspection of the skin, eyes, throat, and nasal passages, and on auscultation of the lungs (see Question 25). An attentive physician can therefore detect various specific findings of allergy if they are present on the physical examination.

Allergists are experts in evaluating and managing children and adults who have allergic diseases.

After obtaining a complete history and performing a physical examination, the next step in the evaluation may on occasion require allergy testing. These tests are performed either directly on the patient (*in vivo*) or as a laboratory procedure (*in vitro*). More information about the different types of allergy testing is presented in the next question as well.

Direct testing involves two similar but slightly different techniques. Allergists usually initially begin testing a child with the "prick-puncture" method which is performed on the skin of the patient's forearm or back. The "prick puncture" form of testing does not involve getting an injection. If the "prick puncture" testing is not definitive, then the next step in the evaluation of suspected allergy may require intradermal tests, typically on the upper arm. A very superficial injection into the skin and no deeper is necessary for an intradermal test. In the hands of a well-trained technician, nurse, or physician, this often-dreaded part of an allergy evaluation should not become a traumatic experience for either the patient or the parent (see Question 34). A positive test indicates that your child has been exposed to a specific allergen (for example, birch tree pollen) and has become "sensitized" to that substance. Your child's immune system has been stimulated to produce a special protein called an antibody, in this case an IgE anti–birch tree antibody. Your child is now "primed" to have an allergic reaction on his next exposure to birch tree pollen.

The potentially confusing aspect of allergy testing is to understand the significance of a positive test. As detailed in the next section (Question 34), your child may have a positive test result but if he or she does not experience allergic symptoms too, then true allergy is not present. A child without symptoms when exposed to an allergen, but who tests positive for that allergen has been "sensitized." Sensitization means that the child has the "potential" to develop allergy symptoms when exposed to that allergen. The good news is that your allergist has the knowledge and experience required to correctly interpret and explain all the data that are collected during an allergy evaluation.

Once the diagnosis of a specific allergy (or allergies) is established, the next step is initiating appropriate treatment. There are three basic and complementary approaches to the treatment of allergic diseases: allergen avoidance, medications, and immunotherapy. The first measure is to avoid contact with and exposure to the allergen whenever that is at all possible. With a food allergy, in particular, complete avoidance of the specific food that causes the allergic reaction is the only way for your child to be safe. Unfortunately, there are some allergens, such as tree pollen, that cannot reasonably be avoided, and others (like the adored family pet) that might be extremely difficult to avoid. Even so, it is also important for a child to have as normal and healthy a lifestyle as possible despite the presence of an allergic condition. If your child is allergic to an environmental allergen (such as a cat, dog, or hamster) and you consistently and reliably implement successful environmental allergen control, your child may not require any further medication or other treatment. However, environmental control alone is unfortunately rarely sufficient in treating childhood allergy (see Question 70). More commonly, despite excellent environmental control and determined efforts at allergen avoidance, additional measures are required for optimal allergy treatment.

The next step in allergy treatment is the prescription of appropriate medications (pharmacotherapy) to effectively control your child's symptoms. Note, however, that the medications prescribed for control of allergy symptoms cannot cure your child of the underlying allergy.

Immunotherapy is the third approach employed for the treatment of allergic asthma. Immunotherapy, which is commonly referred to as "allergy shots," is the only method of treatment that has the potential to turn down, or possibly turn off, the ability of the patient's immune system to react to specific allergens. If there is no allergic reaction, there will be no asthma symptoms.

Consider, for instance, a patient with documented tree and grass pollen allergies whose parents came to us seeking a second opinion when he was 11 years old. He had first developed allergy symptoms in first grade. Over the next four years, and despite excellent compliance with antihistamine pills, nasal allergy sprays, and environmental controls such as use of air conditioning and air filters, this youngster experi-

Environmental control

One of the three components of a comprehensive management and treatment program for children with allergy and asthma. Specifically, the term refers to the avoidance or elimination from the home, school, or work environment of those substances, allergens, or irritants that are responsible for a patient's allergy symptoms.

Pharmacotherapy

Treatment by medication administered either by mouth, through injection, inhalation, or intravenously.

enced worsening allergic symptoms every spring and summer. Immediately before he was brought in for his consultation, he required several courses of oral corticosteroid medication over the course of a single spring and summer season. One of our treatment recommendations included consideration of immunotherapy directed against tree and grass allergens. This patient proceeded with immunotherapy and is now an active, sports-loving 16-year-old who no longer needs to use nasal steroid sprays and daily antihistamines in order to function. During the "allergy season"—spring into early summer—he takes only an infrequent antihistamine to control his almost non-existent symptoms. Participation in his favorite sports— soccer and baseball—no longer presents the challenges it did before he started his allergy treatments. Immunotherapy directed against tree and grass pollens has caused his immune system to turn down and almost turn off his ability to react allergically to either of these pollen classes. With continued therapy, it would not be unreasonable for this young man to be rid of his allergic sensitivity to the spring-season pollens.

Allergists are experts in administering immunotherapy. Immunotherapy has been proven effective in the treatment of selected persons with allergic asthma, allergic rhinitis, and insect sting allergy. Treatment is ongoing for an average of three to five years and initially requires weekly visits. Over time, the interval between injection visits extends to three or four weeks during the maintenance phase. A child who fails to respond satisfactorily to a combination of environmental control measures and drug treatment, may be considered as a potential candidate for immunotherapy.

34. My daughter is very frightened of needles. If I take her to an allergist, what kinds of tests will be done to determine if she is allergic?

Many people have heard "terrible" stories of what happens in an allergist's office. There is a great misconception that everyone who goes to an allergist will be tested with dozens

Diagnostic Evaluation and Workup

Immunotherapy

One of the three main therapeutic approaches to the management of allergic disorders, in which patients are given subcutaneous injections of the specific allergens responsible for their symptoms. The purpose of the treatment is to decrease or eliminate the patient's sensitivity to a given allergen by stimulating the production of a protective (blocking) IgG antibody.

of needles or shots. The most important part of any allergy evaluation is the history that is obtained by your child's physician. The necessity to perform allergy testing depends on your child's individual history.

Many children who go to an allergist do not necessarily require testing. If tests are required, they will be performed either directly or through a blood sample. People mistakenly believe that the allergy blood test (RAST®) is more accurate than direct allergy testing in allergy evaluation. In reality, that is not true. The RAST®, which stands for Radio-AllergoSorbentTest®, is a valid technique for determining allergic sensitivity. Specific clinical situations lead an allergist to recommend the RAST® method of testing. Children who have skin conditions, such as eczema, or very reactive skin are not appropriate candidates for direct allergy testing and are better evaluated with a RAST®. The very young child and one who has an exaggerated fear of needles would be possible candidates for RAST® testing as well. Testing for many different suspected food allergies in a young child can be performed effectively all at once with the RAST® procedure.

Direct allergy testing is a more sensitive technique than the RAST®. Direct testing includes the prick puncture (or "scratch" test) as well as the intradermal test. Prick puncture is generally performed on the inside of the patient's forearm and the intradermal test on the upper arm. When performed by a skillful technician, nurse, or physician, the testing session should not be a traumatic experience for your child.

Why are allergy tests performed at all? In almost all cases, allergy tests should be performed to confirm the allergist's clinical impression derived from a detailed history and physical examination. A positive test result means that your child has the potential to develop symptoms (such as rash, cough, wheeze, sneeze, itch) when exposed to that specific substance or item. A positive allergy test by itself is not an absolute indicator that your child will ever have symptoms. It is necessary to have both a specific positive history of allergic type symptoms and the confirmatory test before a cause-and-effect relationship can be established. The history and corresponding test are like pieces of a puzzle that match. A positive history and a positive test function like a lock and key working together. The history is the lock and the positive allergy test is the key, and together they can open the door to a variety of symptoms. If you only have one without the other, you cannot be certain that an allergic reaction is responsible for your child's symptoms.

There is no question that allergy testing is an important part of your child's complete evaluation, but it should not be the main reason you go to an allergist. An appropriate consultation should consist of five components: history, physical examination, any indicated tests, review of diagnoses, and recommendations for management. In the hands of a skilled professional, a testing session should not be a frightening experience for you or for your child. On the contrary, you should both feel that your child's symptoms are being addressed in a caring, professional, and scientific manner, and that you and your child's doctor will gain useful and practical insights on how best to manage allergy symptoms.

Kerrin's comment:

We had my son tested for allergies when he was 2 years old. We were especially concerned about a peanut allergy because he had a reaction to a cookie someone brought from a bakery that we suspected had either been made with peanut oil or had come in contact with peanut ingredients. The allergy specialist performed a test on his back because he was too young to be certain he would not wipe off the serum. The hardest part was keeping him still for the twenty minutes it took for the test to complete. But they had a VCR in the office and he quickly settled down. And the test showed that he had a severe peanut allergy, so the very short discomfort was a small price to pay for knowing this potentially life-saving piece of information.

35. How does a doctor diagnose asthma?

The diagnosis of asthma is often straightforward, especially for an experienced physician or specialist, but can also be frustrating and elusive. Asthma can manifest differently in different individuals because of its waxing and waning nature and its variability. A physician evaluating a child with a typical, or textbook, presentation will likely be able to correctly diagnose asthma at the first visit. A patient with variant or atypical symptoms may require repeat visits, a trial of asthma medicine, or even specialized diagnostic testing to confirm the diagnosis.

More severe forms of asthma are usually easier to pinpoint and diagnose accurately as compared to less clear-cut presentations. Consider some examples in each category. A previously healthy, nonsmoking teenage girl who reports an episodic history of intermittent wheezing, cough, chest discomfort, and breathlessness with exposure to cold winter air is describing a history typical of asthma. Another youngster, who sees the doctor because of a nagging cough and whose parents are concerned about chronic or recurrent bronchitis and colds, might actually have asthma. Similarly, the athlete who gets really winded playing racquetball and then gets used to coughing for a few hours after each match could certainly have exercise-induced asthma.

Asthma can be confidently diagnosed when specific symptoms, physical examination findings, and specialized test abnormalities are present. The first step in evaluating suspected asthma is a complete medical history, during which the doctor, patient, and parents meet face-to-face for an in-depth conversation and exchange of information. The patient or parents describe the symptoms in detail and as accurately as possible, and the physician asks a series of directed questions regarding lung health, followed by more general health inquiries. In this way, the physician will obtain information not only about the patient's specific pulmonary symptoms but also about the presence or absence of allergies or other medical or surgical conditions. The physician obtains other important background information from reviewing the patient's medication history and their travel, recreational, and social history.

Some questions may seem curious at first, but should nonetheless be answered truthfully. When physicians ask parents if they have wall-to-wall carpeting in the bedroom or who does the vacuuming, for example, they are far from interested in discussing domestic decorating or cleaning arrangements. Rather, they are gathering facts to help decide if an allergic response to the home environment is a possibility. Similarly, when they ask, "Is anyone else at home coughing?" or "Is anyone at home a smoker?", they are searching for clues to help hone in on the correct diagnosis. All conversations between physicians and patients are entirely confidential; truthfulness is an important part of the successful doctor–patient relationship. Just as physicians would never think of telling a patient an untruth, so, too, do they trust their patients and parents to provide an accurate description or history.

After history-taking comes the physical examination. Most lung specialists will perform a directed physical examination, with special emphasis on the respiratory system. One can expect measurement of vital signs, including weight and height, blood pressure, respiratory rate, pulse, and, if necessary, temperature. The lungs are examined by inspection and auscultation. Inspection refers to a visual look; for example, do both lungs move in and out with each breath? Percussion involves gently tapping on the chest. If the lungs are full of air, the tapping will sound "resonant." If they are not filled with air, then the tapping will sound "dull." Auscultation requires a stethoscope. The examiner will ask the patient to inhale and exhale deeply and regularly during auscultation. The presence or absence of wheezing is especially significant, as is the finding of cough, particularly one triggered by inhaling deeply. Other important features of the physical assessment include examination of the eyes, ears, nose, throat, heart, and

Physicians can often suspect the presence of an allergy based on historical information, and detect allergic changes on a careful physical examination.

skin. Although physicians can often suspect the presence of an allergy based on historical information, they can also often detect allergic changes on a careful physical examination.

After the history and physical examination are completed, the doctor will be able to generate a list of diagnostic possibilities, called the *differential diagnosis*. The doctor's clinical impression rates the possible diagnoses in order of likelihood. Sometimes it may be obvious to the doctor that asthma is present. If not, and if asthma is high on the list of possible explanations for a patient's symptoms, then additional diagnostic testing might be considered.

36. What diagnostic tests are available to confirm that my child has bronchial asthma?

The single most helpful diagnostic tests for asthma are pulmonary function tests (PFTs) (discussed in detail in Question 37). PFTs are also used to monitor asthma activity and severity over time, especially in older children and in adults. Other useful tests include blood tests and X-ray studies. Additional, more specialized studies may also be indicated. An example of a specialized study is skin-prick puncture testing for suspected allergy. Assessment of immune function and allergies, for example, can be performed partly through blood testing (discussed in Question 33). Chest X-rays provide information about the anatomy or structure of the lungs and the larger breathing passages. Although chest CT scans are not usually required for the diagnosis and care of children with asthma, they do provide an extremely detailed picture of the lung's appearance or anatomy. In quiescent, controlled asthma, the chest X-ray should be entirely normal. During a marked exacerbation that requires hospital care, for instance, the lungs' appearance on an X-ray may suggest what radiologists call hyperinflation, and a CT might show findings of air trapping. Both findings reflect the uneven lung filling and emptying when breathing occurs through inflamed, constricted air tubes.

37. What is a pulmonary function test? Can my 5-year-old undergo a pulmonary function test?

If your 5-year-old can follow directions and if he is tested by a physician, nurse, or technician knowledgeable in performing pulmonary function tests in children, then yes, your child can undergo the testing.

Pulmonary function tests (PFTs) as the name implies, are designed to measure lung function. PFTs were originally used as research tools, available only in specialized academic hospital centers. At first, they were performed only on adults. Testing is easier to perform on older children and adult subjects who can reliably follow instructions, such as, "Take in the biggest breath you can hold, and then blow out as hard and as rapidly as you can." Studies have shown, however, that experienced technicians or physicians can accurately and reliably obtain pulmonary function testing on children as young as 5 or 6 years of age, thus obtaining accurate measurements of lung function. PFTs are now widely available and are frequently indicated because of their usefulness in diagnosing and treating asthma.

A pulmonary function test measures lung function.

The term "PFT" is used to describe several different specific lung tests (Table 15). Spirometry is the most useful PFT for diagnosing and treating asthma. Spirometry includes two important subtests. The first is called the peak expiratory flow (PEF). The second is the FEV_1, the forced expiratory volume in one second. Measurements of PEF and FEV_1 are thus parts, or subtests, of the spirometry portion of the PFTs. The availability of inexpensive, highly portable, and easy-to-use peak flow monitors makes it possible for every patient with asthma to measure peak flow, at home, on a daily basis. FEV_1 measurements, on the other hand, require the use of a spirometer, which is far more costly, requires special maintenance, and is impractical for home use. Self-monitoring of PEF gives patients with asthma and their parents insight into the condition and allows them to assess their asthma control. Both

FEV_1

Forced expiratory volume in one second, which is a sub-test of the spirometry portion of the pulmonary function tests. Both the FEV_1 and a second measurement, the FEV_1/FVC ratio, are used to diagnose asthma and to assess and follow response to treatment.

PEF and FEV$_1$ play a role in the NAEPP's asthma diagnosis, classification, and treatment guidelines.

Table 15   Pulmonary Function Tests

Pulmonary function tests (PFTs) were originally designed for physiologic lung research. No longer a specialized research tool, PFTs help clinicians establish the diagnosis of asthma and answer practical questions about disease management and treatment. Items in **boldface** are PFTs used in the National Asthma Education and Prevention Program's (NAEPP) asthma classification and treatment guidelines. Spirometry is a commonly used office-based test. PFTs other than spirometry require sophisticated equipment and are performed either in a hospital-based pulmonary laboratory or a pulmonary specialist's office.

Spirometry (includes **FEV$_1$, FEV$_1$/FVC ratio**, and **peak expiratory flow**)
- *Measures how severe asthma is*
- *Measures how active asthma is*
- *Determines how well-controlled asthma is*
- *Determines whether additional medicine is likely to help*

Measurement of Lung Volumes
- *Indicates the largest volume of air the child's lungs can contain*
- *Determines how severe asthma is*

Measurement of Airway Resistance
- *Determines how severe asthma is*
- *Assesses how much resistance air encounters moving through the lungs' breathing passages*

Measurement of Diffusion
- *Abnormal in severe exacerbations*
- *Measures how well oxygen can enter the body through the lungs*

Measurement of Gas Exchange, or Arterial Blood Gas
- *Affected in severe exacerbations*

Bronchoprovocation Studies
- *Determines whether asthma could be the diagnosis, even if all other of the above PFT results are entirely within normal limits*

Note: It is very difficult for children younger than 5 years to reliably perform PFTs and spirometry.

To perform spirometry and PEF, the patient is first asked to take a maximal, deep breath of room air. The biggest single breath is then forcefully and rapidly exhaled into a mouthpiece connected to the spirometer or peak flow meter. The maneuver is repeated several times during testing to ensure accurate, reproducible values. The spirometer measures the entire exhaled lung volume and the flow of air through the mouthpiece during the time that exhalation takes place. The measurements are recorded by the spirometer, printed out, and graphed for review and future reference. Each individual measurement is compared with a predicted value. The predicted values for pulmonary function tests are based on three variables: (1) age, (2) height, and (3) gender. Predicted values for a 16-year-old, six-foot-tall boy are different from those for a four-foot-tall, 7-year-old girl. Therefore, the PEF value or FEV_1 that is considered normal for a short, younger girl with asthma would be abnormal for a tall, adolescent boy with asthma.

Because asthma is characterized as a disease of lung emptying, exhalation time is abnormally prolonged in asthma. Anyone with active asthma who attempts to blow out all the candles on a birthday cake with one single mighty blow of air knows about impaired lung emptying firsthand. Depending on the degree of asthma and other factors, such as how much airway narrowing or bronchospasm is present, full exhalation during spirometry might last as long as twelve to fourteen seconds rather than the normal five to six seconds. The FEV_1 and PEF values reflect the efficiency of lung emptying and thus provide information about how a person's lung function is affected by their asthma.

The FEV_1 is defined as the volume of air that is exhaled in the first second of forceful exhalation as measured using spirometry. If asthma is poorly controlled, the lungs will take longer than predicted to fully empty. Because total exhalation time is prolonged in asthma, the amount or volume of air exhaled in the first second of exhalation is reduced compared with a predicted normal. The FEV_1 will be decreased in symptomatic or poorly controlled asthma. With treatment, the lungs should empty more efficiently and the FEV_1 value should return to normal.

Spirometry in active asthma reveals reduced flow rates. The peak flow is the single greatest value of flow measurement that occurs as the lungs begin to empty after a deep inhalation. Peak flows reflect the flow of air through the larger airways. Peak flow values generally track asthma activity. Home-based PEF monitoring can then help identify even a mild exacerbation and guide medication adjustment up or down, depending on how the PEF value fluctuates from predicted personal best values. Self-administered PEF measurements over time are a component of asthma action plans.

38. Will a chest X-ray help diagnose asthma? Is it necessary to get an X-ray of my child's chest if asthma is suspected?

Chest X-rays provide information about the anatomy or structure of the lungs and larger breathing passages. They are not required in the routine assessment of a child with asthma or for diagnosing asthma, but may be very useful in diagnosing other lung ailments and lung infections.

Asthma is a disease that affects the flow of air through the breathing passages. It does not change the overall appearance or anatomy of the lung structure, and therefore the chest X-ray, or lung picture, should be normal in children with stable controlled asthma. If a child experiences a severe exacerbation or asthma attack requiring hospitalization, then the chest X-ray may reveal changes such as what radiologists call hyperinflation. The finding of hyperinflation on an X-ray reflects the uneven lung filling and emptying when breathing occurs through inflamed, constricted air tubes. The hyperinflation is reversible with treatment of the exacerbation and attack. As the asthma is controlled, the hyperinflation subsides and the chest X-ray normalizes.

39. Are any tests available that can determine how severe my child's asthma will become?

No one test alone can accurately determine the current severity of your child's asthma, and no medical test exists that can predict the future course of your child's asthma. How we would all love to be able to consult a crystal ball that holds all the answers! Asthma is an inherently variable disease. Its manifestations vary from child to child, and in a given child, asthma symptoms and severity can vary over time. Lung function tests (PFTs), repeated periodically, provide objective data that can assist physicians in assessing the severity of your child's asthma and the response to treatment, or the degree of asthma control. Most children over 5 years of age can be taught how to perform pulmonary function tests. Because asthma is such a variable disease, overall assessment of asthma severity and control in an individual child is thus best determined by treatment, observation, clinical monitoring, and testing over an extended period. Part of asthma treatment must include ongoing self-monitoring along with periodic physician reassessments. In particular, if your child's symptoms are well controlled and his asthma is asymptomatic on treatment for three or more consecutive months, consideration of "stepped-down" therapy might then be appropriate and should be considered in consultation with your child's physician.

Statistics about asthma, its severity, and prognosis are derived from in-depth studies of large numbers of persons and provide useful information for medical researchers, public health experts, and policy makers. Statistics about populations cannot, however, be applied to an individual person or patient, such as your child. Consider a nonmedical example. Let's say that a study of all 10-year-olds in an elementary school reveals that 70% of the 10-year-olds have an older sibling. Does that statistical fact mean that your 10-year-old has a 70% chance of having an older brother or sister? Not at all—your child either does or does not have an older sibling, and this is not a phenomenon that can be measured in percentages or statistics.

Asthma is a disease that affects the flow of air through the breathing passages and does not change the overall appearance or anatomy of the lung structure.

Diagnostic Evaluation and Workup

The fact that a majority (70%) of 10-year-olds at school have an older brother or sister, although true, cannot be applied to your child as an individual; the statistic in no way predicts whether your child is or is not an only child.

During episodes of severe asthma requiring emergency room treatment or hospitalization, accurate assessments can be made about the current level of severity of your child's condition. Through close clinical observation and periodically monitoring oxygen levels, electrolyte levels, and pulmonary function tests, your child's status at any point in time can be determined.

40. How will I know if my son's asthma attack is severe enough to require a trip to the emergency room? Are there specific signs and symptoms that can help me make that decision?

Every year children with asthma have attacks and disease exacerbations that are severe enough to require treatment in a hospital emergency department. In 2002, 1.9 million emergency department visits occurred for this purpose. Of this number, more than 700,000 emergency visits were in children aged 17 years and younger. As this statistic shows, you may find yourself seeking medical care in an emergency room for your child who may be out of breath, coughing, or wheezing.

At some point, parents of children who have asthma may have to consider the possibility that they will have to take their child to a hospital emergency room for treatment of a severe asthma attack. It is important to remember that you should not have to make this decision by yourself. Every child who has asthma must have a primary care physician, and many families also have a relationship with either a pulmonologist or an allergist. Frequent communication with the members of your child's medical team will provide you with the assistance to simplify the decision-making process.

The observations you make regarding the pattern of your child's symptoms will enable the doctor to decide if and when you need to go to the hospital. Several physical signs can help you determine if your child's symptoms are reaching the critical point and require treatment available only at an emergency room. His ability to play, eat, and talk, and his respiratory rate (number of breaths per minute), the presence of retractions (sucking in of the spaces between the ribs), and cyanosis (presence of a bluish color involving the lips and the areas under the fingernails) should all be noted. The need for increasingly frequent doses of short-acting, quick-relief β_2 agonist medication, such as albuterol, levalbuterol, or pirbuterol is an ominous sign.

Signs of impending danger consist of a lack of interest in playing, difficulty eating, and increasing difficulty in speaking more than a few words at a time. In the early stages of an asthma exacerbation, you should count the number of times per minute that your child takes a breath (respiratory rate). This will give you a baseline that you can use to monitor the progression of your child's symptoms. An increasing respiratory rate indicates that your child's asthma is worsening. Every breath we take requires a certain physical effort; this reflects the work of breathing. If your child's respiratory rate is increasing, he is working harder and will become very tired as time passes. Once significant fatigue develops, your child's ability to maintain adequate respiration rapidly declines.

Retractions involving the rib cage and the presence of cyanosis are further indications that your child's condition can no longer be managed at home and it is critical that you immediately go to the hospital. Depending on the distance between your home and the hospital, it is sometimes wiser to call 911 for emergency assistance in getting to the emergency room.

The decision to bring your child to the emergency room will depend on many factors; however, the most important is your feeling as a parent that your child requires more help than you

Respiratory rate

Number of breaths per minute.

Retractions

A "sucking in" or visible depression of the muscles in the spaces between the ribs that occurs with labored breathing.

Cyanosis

A bluish discoloration best detected in the nail beds (under the fingernails) and around the lips, indicating abnormally low levels of blood oxygen.

can provide for them at home. It is always wiser to go to the hospital earlier rather than later. It is far better to hear that your child's condition is not as serious as it appeared at first than it is to wait too long and have your child end up in the intensive care unit.

The decision to bring your child to the emergency room will depend on many factors.

Kerrin's comment:

When my son had his first respiratory episode, we didn't know what was happening. He had a cold, he had a very productive-sounding cough, and he was wheezing. We had the nebulizer from an earlier illness he had during which his doctor heard wheezes, although nothing as extreme as what we were hearing this time. We used the nebulizer, which worked for a short time, but only a couple of hours. We had to re-treat him within two hours. We put him to bed after one of the treatments and he seemed to be doing better, but after checking on him an hour later we thought he might be having trouble again. It was hard to tell, though, because he was asleep, we couldn't really see the retractions in his chest, and we thought perhaps his deep breathing was just from the fact that he was asleep. When we called the doctor, she asked us to hold the phone up to his mouth so she could hear him, and she told us to look at his neck to see if retractions were occurring there; they were, and they were very obvious. Hearing this, combined with the fact that we were having to readminister treatments within less than four hours, she told us to take him straight to the hospital. He ended up having to stay for two days.

PART FOUR

Diagnosis and Differential Diagnosis

What specific symptoms should make me suspect that my child has asthma?

Are there any tests that will prove that my child has asthma?

What is the difference between allergy and asthma?

More . . .

41. Are there other conditions that can be confused with asthma because of a similar pattern of symptoms?

A detailed history of the present symptoms is often the best diagnostic tool your pediatrician has to make an accurate diagnosis. For this reason, the information you provide should be as specific as possible. In some situations, the doctor will have to rule out other conditions that can be confused with asthma before arriving at a final diagnosis (see Table 11 in Question 26).

Once the history and physical examination have been performed, the doctor may order several tests to complete the evaluation. The diagnostic options may include allergy tests; lung function tests; chest X-rays; computed tomography (CAT) scans of the sinuses; magnification X-rays of the upper airways; fiberoptic examination (rhinoscopy) of the nose, throat, and vocal cords; pH tests of the esophagus and the sweat; and blood tests. Fortunately, most patients never require such an extensive workup.

Many children begin to wheeze before their first birthday. During the first year, wheezing that develops in association with a respiratory tract infection is not unusual. Bronchiolitis, typically caused by a virus, involves the smallest air passageways (bronchioles) within the lung. As a result of the infection, narrowing of the bronchioles occurs secondary to inflammation and swelling. This sequence of events commonly results in wheezing and respiratory distress.

Tracheomalacia is a condition found in some newborns and is caused by immature development of the cartilaginous rings that provide the framework for the trachea. Infants who have this self-correcting anatomic problem frequently develop inspiratory stridor, a sound heard as the child breathes in (inspiration). Stridor may be mistakenly identified as a wheeze.

A detailed history of a child's present illness is often the best diagnostic tool a pediatrician has to make an accurate diagnosis.

Bronchiolitis

An inflammation of the tiniest bronchial tubes. Bronchiolitis can be secondary to an infection (infectious bronchiolitis) or caused by a noninfectious cause such as cigarette smoking (smoker's bronchiolitis).

Stridor

A high pitched, harsh, vibratory noise caused by partial airway obstruction, which results in turbulent airflow.

Inspiration

The act of taking a breath of air into the lungs. The respiratory cycle has two parts: inspiration and expiration.

In comparison, the typical asthmatic wheeze is audible as a child breathes out (exhales). As children grow, the rings of cartilage in the trachea become stiffer and the symptoms of trachoemalacia eventually disappear. During the first few months of life, congenital anomalies such as vascular rings, laryngeal webs, tracheostenosis, and bronchopulmonary dysplasia can similarly cause breathing difficulty and wheezing. Appropriate imaging studies, including X-ray, MRI, and high-resolution CAT scans, help physicians discover these physical abnormalities. These abnormal anatomic conditions require corrective surgery.

Aspiration of food or other foreign objects into the bronchial passageways may be associated with wheezing. Usually the wheeze is heard only on one side of the chest (unilateral). In this situation, the use of a bronchodilator, such as albuterol, may not provide effective symptom relief. A high index of suspicion, leading to a chest X-ray, will often confirm the diagnosis.

Enlarged tonsils or adenoids may cause nighttime cough and produce sounds that are sometimes confused with a wheeze. This diagnosis should be suspected based on the initial history and physical examination.

Gastroesophageal reflux disease (GERD) is a condition that should be suspected in a child who frequently vomits after eating or who begins to cough after going to bed (see Question 42). An older child who complains of heartburn or discomfort after meals associated with wheezing should be evaluated for GERD. Asthma and GERD frequently coexist; the reflux can aggravate and serve as an asthma trigger. Patients with GERD may require ongoing management with either an otolaryngologist or a gastroenterologist.

Cystic fibrosis may present with symptoms of chronic obstructive lung disease. Children with this serious genetic condition may

Gastroesophageal reflux disease (GERD)

A medical condition that often leads to abdominal symptoms and heartburn, and may also significantly worsen underlying asthma. GERD, or more simply reflux, is usually treated with a combination of dietary changes and medicine.

demonstrate failure to thrive, along with gastrointestinal and lung symptoms. Respiratory symptoms typical of cystic fibrosis include a chronic cough, wheezing, and recurrent pulmonary infections. Cystic fibrosis is classified as a rare disease as it occurs in about one in three thousand births and affects approximately thirty thousand persons in the United States. Not infrequently, bronchial asthma develops in children with cystic fibrosis. When cystic fibrosis is suspected, the diagnosis can be confirmed with appropriate DNA-based testing and a sweat chloride test.

Rhinitis and sinusitis may cause chronic coughing, which usually worsens after a child has gone to sleep. Symptoms of nasal congestion, a postnasal drip, and pain involving the forehead and cheekbones should arouse suspicion of a problem occurring in the nose or the sinuses. If the primary area of involvement is in the sinuses, a CAT scan is a good way for the doctor to visualize the area to confirm the diagnosis. Appropriate medical management, which may include antibiotic therapy, antihistamines, decongestants, saline sinus irrigation, or intranasal steroid sprays, will generally reduce or eliminate the problem.

Vocal Cord Dysfunction Syndrome (VCD)

A condition that can be confused with asthma. VCD's primary disturbance involves the vocal cords and their abnormal tendency to move toward each other (rather than move apart) during inspiration, or breathing in.

Vocal cord dysfunction (VCD) was first described in 1983 at National Jewish Hospital in Denver, Colorado. The condition occurs as a result of abnormal or paradoxical motion of the vocal cords (see Question 42). Normally the vocal cords open and move apart as we breathe air in and out; however, with VCD the cords move together as air is inhaled. This abnormal action causes several symptoms and complaints that may include shortness of breath, a sensation of tightness involving the chest and/or throat, trouble getting air in, and intermittent bouts of persistent wheezing or hoarseness. Patients with VCD usually do not respond to the medications customarily used to treat asthma. Children with this condition make frequent visits to the emergency room for treatment of rapid-onset severe respiratory symptoms. In order for this condition to be diagnosed, it first must be suspected and then confirmed through fiberoptic examination of the vocal cords during an attack. Treatment by a speech pathologist can be very effective in controlling the symptoms of this condition, as further described in Question 42.

Many different medical and surgical conditions may cause symptoms that mimic those of asthma and therefore should be considered in the differential diagnosis of the child who has difficulty breathing and symptoms of cough or wheeze.

42. What is vocal cord dysfunction syndrome (VCD)? What is reflux/GERD, and why does it affect my child's asthma?

Several medical conditions can mimic asthma, and not all of them are lung conditions. Two important medical illnesses that can be confused with asthma are vocal cord dysfunction syndrome (VCD) and gastroesophageal reflux disease (GERD).

VCD is a complex condition characterized by abnormal paradoxical movement of the vocal cords. Normally, the two vocal cords look like a "V." When you take a breath in, the vocal cords assume an even wider "V" shape and spread further apart to allow air into the trachea and lungs. In active VCD, however, the vocal cords close instead of opening during inspiration. Because the cords swing together instead of moving apart, the flow of air into the trachea and lungs becomes compromised. Upper-airway wheezing occurs as air is forced through the abnormally narrowed vocal cord opening. Other symptoms of VCD include a change in voice quality, hoarseness, throat or chest tightness, and uncomfortable swallowing.

Several medical conditions can mimic asthma, and not all of them are lung conditions.

VCD is often misdiagnosed as asthma, especially as difficult-to-control, or refractory, asthma. Clues to its diagnosis include nonresponse to asthma treatment, a preponderance of throat symptoms, and absence of the nocturnal symptomatology characteristic of asthma. VCD can occur in childhood, adolescence, or adulthood, but is more common in people who are in their 20s to 40s. In younger patients, VCD may occur during competitive sports and seems to have an association with a driven or high-achieving personality style. Psychological factors may also be important in adults. Among adult patients, women predominate, as do female health care workers, for reasons that are not well understood.

If VCD is suspected, referral to a specialized center familiar with diagnosis and treatment of VCD should be strongly considered. It is especially important to determine if VCD is present alone or if there is a dual diagnosis of asthma and VCD, because they can occasionally coexist. Treatment of VCD includes discontinuation of any nonindicated medication, particularly corticosteroids. Specialized speech therapy is the mainstay of treatment and is accompanied, when indicated, by relaxation exercises and psychological support.

Caffeine

A compound found naturally in coffee and tea, and added to other beverages such as soda or energy drinks. It is also added some medications, such as those used for treatment of pain or headache. Caffeine is a weak lung bronchodilator and a central nervous system stimulant, and increases mental alertness and wakefulness. Caffeine acts as a mild kidney diuretic, leading to an increase in urine excretion.

GERD is a medical condition related to the regurgitation of stomach acid. It is a very common condition and can be experienced as heartburn and indigestion. Acid refluxing from the stomach can irritate the vocal cords. Hoarseness and a cough akin to throat clearing may ensue. Finally, any acid reaching the uppermost respiratory passages can cause coughing and even wheezing similar to asthma. GERD not only mimics asthma symptoms, but can also worsen asthma. The good news is that GERD is highly treatable. Treatment consists of straightforward dietary and lifestyle modifications and medication to reduce the stomach's acid production. Sometimes measures as simple as avoiding carbonated beverages, fried foods, and caffeine; eating frequent, smaller meals; and not eating for three hours before bedtime are effective in relieving reflux symptoms. Better reflux control will lead to improved asthma control and reduction of asthma symptoms.

43. What specific symptoms should make me suspect that my child has asthma?

A symptom is an abnormal or unusual sensation, experience, or finding. Asthma can cause different symptoms such as wheezing, coughing, breathlessness, or uncomfortable sensations while breathing. The classical symptom of bronchial asthma is a wheezing sound heard when your child breathes out (expiration). The characteristic wheeze is a high-pitched whistling noise. Wheezing in asthma is rarely present only when a child breathes in (inspiration).

With infants, the observation of rapid breathing, difficulty feeding, or grunting sounds while sucking should make you suspicious of a problem involving the respiratory tract, possibly asthma. In young children (especially in those younger than 5 years old), a persistent dry or nonproductive cough may be the primary asthma symptom. Reports of chest tightness or difficulty breathing, associated with fatigue, may also be the presenting asthma symptom in some children. It is also important to recognize that a 2- to 4-year-old who complains that her chest feels funny or hurts, or an older child who stops participating in athletic activities because of chest discomfort may be experiencing symptoms of bronchial asthma. Although asthma is considered a chronic condition, children who have asthma do not always have obvious clinical symptoms. Table 12 in Question 26 outlines situations that are suggestive of asthma. We strongly believe that if you suspect your child is experiencing any symptoms that could perhaps be due to asthma, then you should definitely report those symptoms to your child's doctor. Your child's physician is qualified to assess any information you bring to his attention, and of course, views your child's health as paramount and will undoubtedly want to get all the details from you and your child!

Another point we want you to keep in mind is that in the interval between periods of active asthma symptoms, your child's physical examination may be completely normal and your child may experience no symptoms of asthma at all. Based on the history you and your child provide, a physician may suspect that your child has asthma. If the doctor then evaluates your child for possible asthma when asthma symptoms are not present, the lung exam may be entirely within

Expiration

The action of breathing air out of the lungs, called exhaling. The respiratory cycle has two parts: inspiration and expiration.

normal limits! Your child can have asthma and a normal lung exam. It is thus very useful from a diagnostic perspective for the doctor to then reexamine your child during an asthma flare, when typical symptoms are present as it can confirm the suspected diagnosis of asthma.

44. Are there any tests that will prove that my child has asthma?

There is no single asthma test that can prove that your child has asthma, as discussed in Question 36. A diagnosis of asthma is based upon the presence or absence of specific symptoms (what the patient actually experiences) and the findings (what the doctor discovers). Several tests are useful to doctors for diagnosing asthma. If we had to pick one test that is most useful in children older than 5 years of age, we would choose pulmonary function testing (PFT) (discussed in Question 37), and of the various PFTs, the single most useful one is spirometry.

The diagnosis of asthma is based upon the presence or absence of different symptoms and the findings of the examination.

Occasionally, a child's spirometry and PFTs are entirely normal. If the physician still thinks that asthma is present, a methacholine (Provocholine®)challenge test may be indicated. A methacholine challenge test is a diagnostic test used in evaluating suspected asthma. The methacholine challenge is also used for research purposes to study airway hyperreactivity. Under special circumstances, it plays a role in the clinical arena. It is one example of a class of specialized tests called "bronchoprovocation tests." Cold-air and exercise tests are other forms of bronchoprovocation testing, but are usually not used in clinical practice.

A bronchoprovocation test might be performed in the evaluation of suspected asthma, particularly in adults. It is rarely required, however, for evaluating a child suspected of having asthma and is not considered a routine test. Bronchoprovocation testing is indicated to further evaluate for the possibility of asthma when: the patient describes subtle symptoms suggestive of asthma or atypical asthma symptoms and spirometry and other pulmonary function testing are entirely normal and when history, physical examination, blood tests, and X-rays do not reveal an alternative diagnosis or medical explanation for the reported symptoms. It is an extremely powerful test for eliminating or "ruling out" asthma. In other words, if the test is negative, asthma is not present. A positive methacholine test result is diagnostic of airway hyperresponsiveness. If the test is thus positive and the symptoms fit, the patient probably has asthma. People with asthma show an increased sensitivity to the inhalation of methacholine, and therefore have positive test results. The converse statement is not true: although everyone with asthma has a positive result on methacholine testing, not everyone who has a positive result has asthma.

The actual methacholine challenge test is usually performed in a hospital pulmonary function laboratory. The test involves obtaining a baseline spirometry measurement and then repeating spirometry after inhalation of higher and higher concentrations of methacholine. The baseline spirometry values should be normal, which is why the challenge test is indicated. If the spirometry measurements remain close to baseline values after inhalation of increasing doses of methacholine, the test is negative and asthma is effectively ruled out. However, if the spirometry values decline significantly after the methacholine inhalation or if wheezing or other symptoms develop, the test is reported as positive. At that point, the testing stops immediately and an inhaled, short-acting bronchodilator is administered to relieve symptoms and reverse the abnormal lung function.

45. Is it true that asthma cannot be diagnosed until my child is older than 2 or 3 years old?

Many children will wheeze during their first twelve months of life; however, only a small percentage of them will ultimately develop asthma. The major trigger for wheezing in the toddler stage is typically a viral respiratory tract infection. When a child has a strong immediate family history of allergy or asthma, especially on the maternal side, he or she has an increased risk for developing bronchial asthma (Table 16).

Table 16   Patterns of Wheezing in Infants

Nonallergic Wheezing
  • Wheezing primarily triggered by viral upper respiratory tract infections
  • Eczema and food allergies are not generally present
  • Wheezing frequently disappears as the baby grows into the pre-school years (3 to 6 years)

Wheezing seen in these infants is not a harbinger of persistent asthma.

Allergic Wheezing
  • Maternal history of asthma or allergy
  • Wheezing develops in association with viral upper respiratory tract infection
  • Allergies such as eczema, food allergy, and rhinitis are often also present
  • Wheezing with viral upper respiratory infections persists as the child grows

The wheezing in these children is likely a symptom of asthma and is likely to become a chronic condition.

A child with a recurring pattern of cough or wheeze that responds to treatment with a bronchodilator (such as albuterol) has bronchoconstriction (tightening of the muscles around the bronchial passageways). Hyperreactivity or hyperirritability of the bronchial passageways is a constant physiologic finding in children who have asthma. We do not know with certainty what factor or factors are necessary to initiate and perpetuate this abnormal response pattern in the lung. Several factors, including genetic, environmental, and infectious, have been identified and may ultimately provide the answer to this question.

It is difficult to be certain that a child has asthma before the age of 18 to 24 months. This is not to say that children younger than that do not develop asthma, only that it is not easy to make a definitive diagnosis at that time. Unless your child has a history of at least three episodes of wheezing, which responded to appropriate pharmacotherapy, experts will be hesitant to make asthma the diagnosis. No blood tests are available that will help confirm the presence of asthma. There is also no readily available method for obtaining lung function studies in children younger than 5 years. For practical purposes, the diagnosis of bronchial asthma in a very young child is generally based on a recurring pattern of cough and/or wheeze that initially respond to a bronchodilator and is controlled long-term with anti-inflammatory drugs. A definitive diagnosis of asthma is also more likely in children under the age of 3 years if the child has experienced more than three episodes of wheezing in the prior twelve months, if the child has a confirmed diagnosis of eczema (atopic dermatitis) and/or allergic rhinitis, if there is a parental history of asthma, and if wheezing has occurred in the absence of a cold or infection.

Kerrin's comment:

I recall being very frustrated by the fact that no one would or could diagnose my son with asthma with certainty before he was about 2 years old. Only after he had three episodes of respiratory difficulty did I hear the word asthma mentioned with conviction. As a parent, you want to know exactly what is happening with your child so that you can be educated and prepared, but without a definite diagnosis of anything, I constantly felt very anxious about his health. After he was finally diagnosed, we were able to educate ourselves about the condition and begin preventive treatment plans.

46. Our 5-year-old coughs whenever she plays outdoors in the snow. My wife is concerned about the cough. I, on the other hand, believe that that we should let our daughter have a good time and forget about the cough. What is the significance of the cough?

Children need exercise and benefit greatly from play and from being outdoors. The presence of cough however is always abnormal.

There are many reasons why cough develops. Cough is a fundamentally protective mechanism that the human body developed to help keep the airways free of mucus and infection. Each one of us has experienced a cough at some point in our lives, such as when ill with a respiratory infection or a head cold. Most coughs caused by colds are short-lived. When a cough lasts for more than two or three weeks or develops in a particular pattern, such as on inhalation of cold air when playing in the snow, take note. Most, but not all, chronic coughs lasting at least six weeks have one or more of three causes: asthma, gastric reflux, or sinus disease. Cough that regularly occurs with exercise, particularly aerobic activities, or cold air exposure strongly suggests the presence of asthma unless proven otherwise.

Once they are properly diagnosed and correctly treated, all children and young people with asthma should be able to participate fully in sports without experiencing asthma flares and should be encouraged to engage in regular exercise.

Exercise is considered a universal trigger for people with asthma. The same is true for cold air exposure. Exercise does not "cause" the condition known as asthma but does lead to increased airway inflammation and acts as a stimulus for bronchoconstriction in people with asthma. Particularly in young children, cough with exertion or exposure to cold should never be ignored; it may be the clue to the diagnosis of asthma. Also remember that regular exercise is a component of modern asthma therapy. Once they are properly diagnosed and correctly treated, all children and young people with asthma should be able to participate fully in sports without experiencing asthma flares and should be encouraged to engage in regular exercise.

47. What is the difference between asthma and allergy?

Asthma and allergy are two different medical conditions. Although they can appear superficially similar and frequently coexist in an individual child, they are best viewed as two entirely separate diagnoses. A 7-year-old boy who is allergic to fish or peanuts, for instance, does not necessarily also have asthma. The same is true for a people who are allergic to a medication, such as penicillin; although they may have an allergy, they do not necessarily have asthma. On the other hand, a 15-year-old girl with asthma who is also allergic to ragweed and experiences increased cough, mucus, chest tightness, and wheezing accompanied by a need to step up her asthma medicines every year in the late summer when airborne ragweed counts are elevated has both asthma and allergy. The boy has a diagnosis of allergy alone, whereas the girl has a dual diagnosis of asthma and allergy, with a specific allergen (ragweed) acting as an asthma trigger.

The term allergy is derived from the Greek words *allos* (other) and *ergeon* (action). An allergy or an allergic reaction is an "other action" or an abnormal response to common substances, such as foods, pollens, or household pets that ordinarily do not cause any reactions at all in other individuals. Most people, for instance, do not sneeze or develop an itchy nose or tearing eyes when there is an elevated pollen count during the spring months, and others never develop swelling of the lips or break out in hives after eating peanuts. People who do develop these reactions are considered to be allergic to tree pollen and peanuts respectively.

Allergic reactions can involve almost any area of the body. Some allergic children develop eczema (atopic dermatitis) or hives (urticaria), others may experience a runny nose and sneezing (allergic rhinitis), and some may have gastrointestinal symptoms such as vomiting and diarrhea. Still others may have reactions involving the lungs and respiratory system with symptoms of cough and wheeze (bronchial asthma). If your child begins to cough and wheeze after playing with the family dog, it would be correct to say that his asthma became symptomatic because of an allergic reaction to the dog dander. In this example, your child, through continued exposure, has become allergic to the family pet, and contact with the dog dander triggers the development of his asthma symptoms.

Urticaria

Hives, a type of skin rash. Hives, or urticaria, are raised, welt-like, reddened, and intensely itchy. The most common cause of urticaria is an allergic reaction. Sometimes, urticaria are idiopathic, meaning that no cause can be identified. Urticaria are treated with anti-inflammatory agents or antihistamines, or both.

In another example, your next-door neighbor's daughter Sally has been diagnosed with asthma. However, the only time she ever wheezes is when she has a respiratory tract infection. When Sally visits your house and plays with your dog, Sally has a great time, feels well, and never experiences any asthma symptoms. Sally has asthma, her asthma symptoms are triggered by viral infections but not by any allergy to your dog.

These two examples illustrate the fact that asthma can occur in children, whether or not they are allergic. Many children and adolescents with asthma are also allergic and may have allergic triggers for their asthma. According to published studies, 60% to 80% of children with asthma are allergic. Note too that some children have both allergic and nonallergic triggers that cause them to develop asthma symptoms, such as breathlessness, cough, increased mucus production, chest tightness, and wheezing (see Question 14). A respiratory infection is an example of a nonallergic trigger, whereas exposure to dog dander is an example of an allergic trigger. Other people with asthma, including many with adult-onset asthma, have no allergies and thus no allergic triggers. The fact is that any individual can have asthma, allergy, or both together. Another fact is that although they are two different and separate diseases, asthma and allergy have much in common.

Symptoms of asthma always arise in the lungs and breathing passages (see Question 1). Symptoms of allergy, on the other hand, certainly can involve the lungs and breathing passages, but can also affect many other organs, such as the skin (hives, urticaria), nasal passages (rhinitis), intestines (food allergies), and eyes (allergic conjunctivitis). Therefore, the lungs are one of many potential targets for allergic symptoms, and asthma can be one particular manifestation of allergy. A key practical concept ensues: the medical evaluation of a child with asthma must include consideration of coexisting allergy. The treating physician should ask questions to assess the likelihood that allergy is playing a role in the child's asthma. If there is a strong probability that allergic triggers are present, further evaluation may assist in pinpointing the specific allergens (see Question 31). An appropriate treatment plan will be formulated to control, eliminate, or neutralize these triggers once they have been identified. Controlling the allergic component of childhood asthma is an important treatment goal.

PART FIVE

Treatment

What medications are helpful for asthma?

What are possible side effects of inhaled
and oral steroids?

How do asthma medicines work?

More . . .

48. What is the National Asthma Education and Prevention Program (NAEPP)? What are the guidelines, and how do they relate to my child's asthma?

The National Asthma Education and Prevention Program (NAEPP) was founded in March 1989 to address the growing problem of asthma in the United States. Although much had been learned about asthma itself, treatment and outcomes were clearly suboptimal, especially when viewed from a national perspective. The NAEPP's primary goal is to improve asthma care in the United States. Its main focus is education: to teach health professionals, asthma patients, and the general public about asthma. The program strives to improve the quality of life of people with asthma, and hopes to decrease asthma-related morbidity and mortality. The NAEPP is administered and coordinated by the U.S. Department of Health and Human Services' National Institute of Heath's National Heart, Lung, and Blood Institute (NHLBI).

The NAEPP's primary goal is to improve asthma care in the United States.

The NHLBI convened a panel of medical experts to improve the clinical management of asthma in the United States and stimulate additional research on asthma (Table 17). Their landmark findings, *Expert Panel Report: Guidelines for the Diagnosis and Management of Asthma,* appeared in 1991. Since then, updated guidelines for diagnosing and treating asthma have been published, reflecting the tremendous amount of new information about asthma. The *Expert Panel Report 2* was published in April 1997. A preliminary draft of the *Expert Panel Report 3* was prereleased on the Internet in February 2007 and the finalized version of the NAEPP *Expert Panel Report 3* should to be available and disseminated by mid to late 2007.

Table 17   Childhood Asthma Treatment Goals/NHLBI Goals of Therapy

Daytime symptoms should be absent or minimal.
Nocturnal symptoms should be absent or minimal; sleep should be restful and uninterrupted.
Absences from work or school because of asthma should be eliminated; parents of children with asthma should similarly not have any missed days of work because of their child's asthma.
Children should experience full participation in sports and athletic competitions with no limitations of activities; regular aerobic exercise is an important component of good asthma management as well as a key feature of a healthy lifestyle for all ages.
Exacerbations should be nonexistent or "few and far between." They should be addressed and treated promptly and effectively. Hospitalizations, asthma emergencies, and emergency room visits should be absent or minimal.
Requirement for fast-acting, quick-relief treatment, usually in the form of a quick-relief, short-acting inhaled β_2 agonist (inhaled or oral, in the case of young children), should be nil or minimal.
Medicines used to treat asthma should be associated with minimal, if any, side effects.
Parents and older children should understand both the written asthma action plan and the emergency asthma action plan.
Children and their parents should expect to visit the treating clinician for asthma follow-up at regular intervals. Visits may need to be scheduled as frequently as monthly or as infrequently as twice a year depending on the level of asthma control. A three-month interval is recommended for children with well-controlled asthma in whom a "step down" in therapy is under way.

In June 2002, the NAEPP provided an additional refinement to the 1997 document: *Expert Panel Report: Guidelines for the Diagnosis and Management of Asthma—Update on Selected Topics 2002*. The expert panel reports are available online through the Internet *(http://www.nhlbi.nih.gov/about/naepp/index.htm* or *http://www.nhlbi.nih.gov/guidelines/asthma/index.htm)* and in print (NHLBI Information Center, P.O. Box 30105, Bethesda, MD 20824-0105). The latest 2007 update includes a modification of the original NAEPP asthma classification along with information on asthma medications and best approaches to treatment. *The Expert Panel Report 3* update emphasizes assessment of asthma severity (as in the prior reports) at the time of asthma diagnosis and adds a complementary assessment of the degree of asthma control obtained through treatment over time. The emphasis on asthma control and response to therapy is a new feature. The latest NAEPP report presents treatment recommendations based on both the initial asthma severity rating as well as on a child's particular response to ongoing treatment or degree of control achieved. The report advocates a six-step approach to the pharmacologic management of asthma and provides detailed treatment suggestions for all children with asthma based on severity, control, and age. *The Expert Panel Report 3* thus separates pediatric patients into three groups for purposes of assessment and asthma treatment: (1) children younger than 5 years of age, (2) children between the ages of 5 and 11 years old, and (3) young people older than 12 years. Within each of those age-related categories, it makes specific treatment recommendations for each level of asthma severity/control and outlines specific medicines for each of the six steps of asthma treatment.

A key component of the NAEPP's asthma treatment guidelines is the classification of asthma into four categories of asthma severity based on symptoms, pulmonary function test values (only in children 5 years old and up), and the need for short-acting, quick-relief β_2 medication to keep symptoms at bay. A child with asthma will fall into one of the four groups at the initial assessment. The guidelines emphasize that once asthma treatment is initiated and continued over time, asthma symptoms should become absent or minimal; so the NAEEP thus believes that assessment of asthma control is an important part of contemporary asthma management and follow-up. Similarly, assessment of asthma control is crucial to identifying a child whose asthma fails to satisfactorily respond to treatment. *The Expert Panel Report 3* provides specific suggestions about how often a child with asthma should be seen in asthma follow-up by their treating doctor. *The Expert Panel Report 3* also provides a framework for assessment of asthma control at those follow-up visits and details when and how to reduce or step down medicines when a child's asthma becomes well controlled as well as how to step-up therapy for the child whose asthma is not well controlled or very poorly controlled.

Patients with asthma can experience exacerbations, which can be mild, moderate, or severe. The importance of correctly assessing and classifying a person's asthma is part of the NAEPP's effort to ensure better care for asthma patients. The NAEPP recommends one of six specific treatments and interventions for each level of asthma severity (Figure 4).

The NAEPP's expert panel classifies four categories of asthma severity. Specific therapies are recommended for each category of asthma.

INTERMITTENT

PERSISTENT
Mild
Moderate
Severe

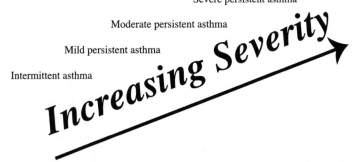

Figure 4   NAEPP's asthma classification.

49. What are the classifications of asthma severity and asthma control according to the National Asthma Education and Prevention Program (NAEPP)?

The NAEPP classifications of asthma severity and asthma control tools were designed to assist clinicians to better care for their patients with asthma and to help patients and their parents participate in ongoing, day-to-day asthma management. The NAEPP classifies asthma severity as (1) intermittent (Table 1 in the appendix, A-1), (2) mild persistent (Table 2 in the appendix, A-2), (3) moderate persistent (Table 3 in the appendix, A-3), or (4) severe persistent (Table 4 in the appendix A-4). The 2007 *Expert Panel Report 3* of the NAEPP introduces for the first time an additional asthma management tool: assessment of asthma control. The degree of asthma control falls into one of three groups: "well controlled," "not well controlled," and "very poorly controlled" which mirror the GINA schema (of "controlled," "partly controlled," and "uncontrolled") as outlined in Question 50.

The 1997 and 2002 NAEPP classifications of four degrees of asthma severity derive from a careful physician assessment of symptoms, need for medication, and the results of pulmonary function testing. Pulmonary function testing is impractical in children less than 5 years of age, so physicians must rely on reports of the frequency of a young child's asthma symptoms, presence and frequency of nighttime awakenings, and the need for short acting β_2 agonist use (needed to maintain symptom control) for severity classification of their youngest asthmatics.

The older NAEPP asthma severity classifications required measurement of either peak expiratory flow (PEF) or forced expiratory volume in one second (FEV_1), whereas the newer ones rely on spirometry (for measurement of FEV_1 for older kids and FEV_1/FVC for ages 5 to 11 years). Both classifications help physicians determine the best initial treatment for children with asthma by suggesting a logical stepwise approach.

The second component—measurement of the extent and success of asthma control—lets doctors determine if ongoing treatment has been effective and efficacious. If so, the 2007 *Expert Panel Report 3* of the NAEPP suggests when and how to step down medications. The guidelines conversely comment on when and how to step up treatment.

50. Are there ways other than the National Asthma Education and Prevention Program (NAEPP) classification to categorize asthma?

Yes, several alternative classifications have recently been developed. They all acknowledge the fact that NAEPP classification has been extremely useful in guiding asthma care and treatment, and has been widely used by practicing physicians in daily patient care.

In May 2006, a task force sponsored by the National Heart, Lung, and Blood Institute; the American Thoracic Society; and the American Academy of Allergy, Asthma, and Immunology unveiled a classification designed specifically for purposes of asthma research. The joint effort divides all asthma into four categories (phenotypes): (1) infection-induced asthma, (2) allergic asthma, (3) nonallergic asthma, and (4) aspirin-sensitive asthma.

Of the four classes, allergic asthma tends to begin early in life and is undoubtedly the most common, affecting up to 88% of all persons with asthma. Infection-induced asthma occurs in children and adults. Nonallergic asthma is more common in adults, and more often in women. Aspirin-sensitive asthma phenotype, a more unusual variant of asthma, affects no more than 5% of childhood asthmatics. The American Thoracic Society believes that the "four phenotype" asthma classification will, according to the American Thoracic Society,

Aspirin

Any preparation of acetylsalicylic acid. Aspirin has analgesic, antipyretic, and anti-inflammatory properties; it is prescribed to relieve pain and fever, rheumatoid arthritis, juvenile rheumatoid arthritis, and many forms of heart disease. Its use is contraindicated in any person with aspirin-sensitive asthma in whom it may trigger wheezing and bronchospasm (exacerbation).

"enhance interpretation of study findings, promote appropriate comparisons among studies, and facilitate genetics research." Time will tell how useful the tool will be.

Nonallergic asthma is more common in adults, and more often in women.

In November 2006, the Global Initiative for Asthma, or GINA, announced the release of its new "Global Strategy for Asthma Management and Prevention." GINA, formed in 1993, works with healthcare professionals worldwide to reduce asthma prevalence, morbidity, and mortality. It began as a collaborative effort between the U.S. National Heart, Lung, and Blood Institute (NHLBI) and the World Health Organization (WHO). GINA is comprised of networks of individuals and organizations committed to asthma care. It maintains a Web site at *www.ginasthma.com* and has sponsored an annual World Asthma Day, held since 1998 on the first Tuesday in May. The new GINA (November 2006) guidelines supplant the GINA statements published in 2002 and are based on a new, easy-to-implement classification of asthma. Previous guidelines (including the 1991, 1997, and 2002 NAEEP) presented asthma management strategies based solely on disease severity. The newer guidelines also take the patient's response to therapy into account and accordingly create a classification based on how effectively the patient's asthma is controlled. The 2006 GINA report (Table 18) thus defines asthma control and bases treatment recommendations directly on its classification of three levels of control: (1) Controlled, (2) Partly Controlled, and (3) Uncontrolled asthma (Table 19). GINA recommends that the previous asthma classification of Intermittent, Mild Persistent, Moderate Persistent, and Severe Persistent not be entirely abandoned, and that it be used for research purposes rather than direct patient care.

Table 18   GINA 2006 Classification and Guidelines: Key Points

Overall, asthma severity is a function of both the severity of the underlying disease and its responsiveness to treatment.

Asthma is classified into one of three (3) categories, based on the level of disease control:

Controlled

Partly Controlled

Uncontrolled

The goal of asthma treatment is to achieve and maintain clinical control.

Treatment of an individual's asthma is based on their level of asthma control.

Treatment options are organized into five "steps" that reflect the intensity of treatment required to obtain asthma control. A reliever medication is part of all steps, and medications of the controller class are part of Steps 2–5.*

Asthma treatment should be adjusted on a continuously based level of asthma control: treatment should be stepped up when control is lost and brought back down when control is achieved.

The severity of a person's asthma may change over time, and the level of control may vary over time as well.

The goal of treatment and the definition of asthma control is:
- No more than twice a week for daytime symptoms
- No limitation of exercise, or of daily activities
- No nocturnal awakenings (or symptoms) because of asthma
- No more than 2× a week need for reliever treatment
- Normal (or near-normal) lung function results
- No exacerbations or asthma "attacks"

*Note that the NAEPP differs slightly as it uses 6 steps of asthma treatment. Reliever medication is part of all steps, and medications of the controller class are part of Steps 2–6 in the NAEPP.

Treatment

111

Table 19   GINA Classification: Levels of Asthma Control

Characteristic	Controlled	Partly Controlled	Uncontrolled
Daytime symptoms	None, to twice or less a week	More than twice a week	Three or more features of partly controlled asthma present in any one-week period classifies asthma as uncontrolled.
Limitation of activities	None	Any limitation	
Nocturnal symptoms or awakenings	None	Any symptom	
Need for reliever (fast-acting) treatment	None, to twice or less a week	More than twice a week	
Lung function* (PEF or FEV$_1$)	Normal	< 80% predicted or than personal best	
Exacerbations	None	One or more a year	One in any week**

*Applies only to children 5 years of age and older as lung function measurements are not considered reliable in younger children and toddlers.

**An exacerbation in any week makes that week an "uncontrolled" asthma week.

51. What is the difference between a medicine's generic and brand name?

All medicines have at least four different names. When a drug is first discovered, it is given a chemical name that describes the molecular composition of the drug. Chemical names are complicated and cumbersome, with parentheses and subscripts, numbers and initials. The pharmaceutical company working to develop the drug for market usually will give the drug an in-house or code name. The name usually includes letters abbreviating the company's name (for example, MSD for Merck or GSK for GlaxoSmithKline), followed by a number. After approval by the U.S. Food and Drug Administration (FDA), the ready-for-market medication is given both a generic and a trade name. Each generic and trade name must be unique and distinctive enough to avoid confusion with other products. In the United States, the United States Adopted Names (USAN) Council assigns a drug its generic name. For example, the generic name for a widely prescribed, quick-relief, fast-acting, short-acting inhaled β_2 agonist medicine is albuterol sulfate. A medicine's generic name is also its official name. The drug's manufacturer then selects the medicine's trade (or brand) name. The FDA must approve the trade name selected by the manufacturer. To use our previous example, the albuterol sulfate inhaler manufactured by the Schering Company is named Proventil® HFA, whereas the inhaler produced by GlaxoSmithKline is Ventolin® HFA. Trade names are often selected to be catchy and easily remembered. The trade name may also reflect a characteristic of the medicine. Many respiratory medicines incorporate "air" or "vent" (as in "ventilation") as part of the trade name. Examples include Singulair®, Advair®, Aerobid®, Maxair®, Xolair®, Flovent®, Serevent®, Atrovent®, Combivent®, Ventolin® HFA, and Proventil® HFA.

When a new medicine is discovered, its inventor applies for a patent for the discovery. The patent details the discovery and, in doing so, makes it public and open to all (including competitors) while protecting the inventor's right to make, use, or sell the medicine for a defined period, after which the patent expires. When a medicine is new on the market and its manufacturer is the only producer of that medicine, only one form of the drug is available to the consumer. Eventually, however, the patent protection expires and other companies may choose to produce the generic form of the medicine. In most cases, the generic form of a medication sold in the United States is pharmacologically equivalent to the brand formulation. Most generic medicine sold in the United States generally costs less than the brand-name medicine and is of good quality. In the state of New York, for example, where we practice allergy and pulmonary medicine, the pharmacist will dispense a generic formulation of the medication we prescribe for our patients unless we specifically write "DAW (dispense as written)" on the prescription. Similarly, your physician will, in most circumstances, have to approve that a prescription medicine be filled with a specific brand rather than a generic formulation.

It is easy to become confused by the fact that a medicine will be called by different names. We usually ask parents and patients to bring all their medicines with them to the office so that we can make sure they understand what medicines they should take and how to take them. We frequently encounter patients who think that they are taking a lot of medicine, only to discover that the two separate inhalers they are using are different only because two different manufacturers are producing the same medicine. If a patient is using inhaled Proventil® HFA along with inhaled Ventolin® HFA, they are really only using one type of drug: the trade form of albuterol sulfate. Remember that the generic name of a medicine refers to the drug itself, whereas the trade name refers to a specific company's product and brand. For example, aspirin is a generic product; Bufferin® is not.

To find out the names of your child's medicines, ask the doctor or pharmacist, and read labels and package inserts. With an inhaled medication, the inhaler label will always carry the drug's trade name along with its generic name, although usually in smaller print. Even over-the-counter medicines are carefully labeled to specify generic and trade names. A final label reading trick to remember is that a trade name is always followed by the ® or ™ symbol, whereas the generic name is not.

52. What medications are helpful for treating asthma?

Many different classes of medicines are useful in treating childhood asthma (Table 20). The asthma classification from the National Asthma Education and Prevention Program (NAEPP) helps define the severity of a person's asthma, assesses response to treatment, and guides therapy. For each asthma classification, the NAEPP makes specific suggestions about the best type of medicine to use for treating that specific level of asthma. Similarly, the more recent GINA classification offers treatment recommendations based on a person's level of asthma control.

Table 20   Medications Used in Asthma Treatment: Classification

Long-Term Daily Control Medications ("Quiet Medications")	Quick-Relief, Fast-Acting Medications ("Noisy Medications")
Inhaled corticosteroids • beclomethasone proprionate • budesonide • ciclesonide • flunisolide • fluticasone • mometasone furoate • triamcinolone acetonide	Inhaled short-acting β_2 agonists • albuterol • levalbuterol • pirbuterol • terbutaline
Mast cell stabilizers • cromolyn sodium • nedocromil sodium	Inhaled anticholinergics • ipratropium bromide
Oral leukotriene modifiers • zafirlukast • zileuton • montelukast	Oral corticosteroids • methylprednisolone • prednisone • prednisolone
Long-acting β_2 agonists • salmeterol • formoterol	
Oral theophylline • sustained release theoplylline	
Emerging therapies • IgE blockers	

Asthma medicines are generally prescribed in a step-wise approach. The physician will begin by prescribing one type of medicine and add or reduce the amount of medication based on the patient's symptom control, lung function, and overall state of well-being. A 10-year-old child with mild intermittent asthma that is well controlled, for example, might be instructed to use a short-acting β_2 inhaler bronchodilator as needed for symptom relief. With the onset of winter and colder temperatures, that child's symptoms may start to increase and become more prominent. The inhaled, short-acting β_2 medicine that formerly kept asthma symptoms under control is now required several times daily to achieve the same level of asthma control. The child's asthma is no longer well controlled and, in fact, has become very poorly controlled. Just as the classification of control has moved up, the treatment is stepped up. Therefore, for a child who previously had mild intermittent controlled asthma, and develops increasing wheezing that is not easily controlled with the use of a short-acting β_2 inhaler, additional medication is required. The child might, for instance, be prescribed a brief "burst" of oral corticosteroid medication along with an inhaled medication with anti-inflammatory properties, such as an inhaled corticosteroid. After a specified amount of time with good asthma control is achieved, a medication step-down can be considered, especially if the reasons for the stepped-up asthma have resolved (such as the end of cold winter weather). Asthma treatment plans must take into account the often fluid and changeable character of asthma itself, along with an individual child's response to medications.

Asthma treatment plans must take into account the often fluid and changeable character of asthma itself.

One method of classifying asthma medicines is by their method of action. The schema includes the major categories of (1) quick-relief, fast-acting bronchodilator medicines, sometimes called "noisy medicines," which are administered as needed to treat noisy symptoms such as wheezing and breathlessness, (2) long-term control medicines taken daily for maintenance of asthma control. These are sometimes called "quiet medicines," since they are designed to be taken daily even though asthma symptoms are controlled or "quiet," and (3) those medicines used to treat an attack or exacerbation.

Metered-dose inhaler (MDI)

Devices that allow the delivery of a precise and accurate dose of medicine to the lungs through inhalation. MDIs are reliable, portable, and very convenient. Many different types of respiratory medicines come in MDI form, including short-acting bronchodilators, inhaled steroids, and anti-inflammatory medicines, as well as inhaled anticholinergics.

Quick-relief, fast-acting bronchodilator asthma medicines are usually inhaled. Even very young children can use inhaled medication (Table 21). Inhaled quick-relief asthma medicines are delivered through metered-dose inhalers (MDIs) or by jet nebulizer. A spacer device or holding chamber attaches to the mouthpiece of an MDI and allows even young children to benefit from the administration of inhaled asthma drugs through an MDI. The inhaled route is preferred because the medicine is delivered directly into the breathing passages. Side effects, if any, are minimal. Why should a child take a medicine in pill form, which leads to measurable drug levels in the entire body, when effective asthma medicine can be deposited exactly where it's needed for a fast action and quick relief of symptoms?

Table 21   Inhaler Devices for Children

Child's Age	Preferred "First Choice"	Alternative Device*
Younger than 4 years	MDI + spacer with face mask	Nebulizer with facemask
4–6 years old	MDI + spacer with mouthpiece	Nebulizer with mouthpiece
Older than 6 years	DPI or Breath actuated MDI or MDI + spacer with mouthpiece	Nebulizer with mouthpiece

MDI = pressurized metered-dose inhaler

DPI = dry powder inhaler.

*Nebulizers are mainly reserved or children who cannot use other inhaler devices

(Adapted from the 2006 GINA *Global Strategy for Asthma Management and Prevention*)

Short-acting β_2 bronchodilator agents, such as albuterol, pirbuterol, levalbuterol, or terbutaline in inhaled form, are all good examples of ideal fast-acting, quick-relief medicines. Quick-relief inhalers are usually prescribed to be taken only when needed. They should be taken at the first sign of asthma symptoms, and are sometimes prescribed before exercize or sports. Their onset of action is rapid and the beneficial effects last between four to six hours. Children should keep their prescribed quick-relief inhaler handy during the day. A school-aged child can keep it in a book bag, purse, pocket, or backpack. School-age children must have reliable and prompt access to their inhalers in school at all times. Like a house key and wallet, a quick-relief inhaler should accompany older children wherever they go.

Treatment

Nebulizer

A device that transforms a respiratory drug in liquid form into a fine mist of medicine particles that are easily inhaled into the respiratory passages. It is powered by a machine or compressor that uses electrical current or batteries. Nebulizers are used for treatment in babies and very young children with asthma who cannot use an MDI or DPI. They are also often used in an emergency setting.

Spacer

A device that facilitates the inhalation of medicine from a metered-dose inhaler (MDI). Spacers allow one to space the required steps for correct MDI use over time. Spacers make it easier to use the MDI medicine, enhance medication delivery to the lungs, and reduce deposition of medicine on the voice box.

Asthma medications used for long-term disease control are asthma medications taken every day to keep asthma under control on a long-term basis. Daily-use or maintenance medicines are used in addition to quick-relief medicine to treat the persistent forms of asthma and those labeled as poorly or not well controlled and uncontrolled. Daily medicines are available in tablet form taken by mouth as well as in inhaled formulations. Inhaled corticosteroids are by far the most effective daily medicines currently available. Inhaled corticosteroids are prescribed either in low, medium, or high dosages depending upon the patient and the extent of asthma control. Inhaled corticosteroids are part of asthma management of steps 2 through 6 of the six step asthma treatment schema advocated by the 2007 NAEPP *Expert Panel 3*. The NAEPP and the GINA recommend inhaled steroids as first-line anti-inflammatory treatment, and advocates their use beginning with mild persistent asthma and with any form of less than completely controlled asthma.

Leukotriene modifiers are a newer class of daily medication approved by the U.S. Food and Drug Administration for young children in addition to adolescents and adults. The leukotriene modifiers seem to be most useful in asthmatics with allergic symptoms, especially if allergic rhinitis coexists with asthma. Leukotriene modifiers are also effective in treating exercise-induced asthma.

Long-term asthma medication must be taken as prescribed, every day, even if symptoms are absent. It is extremely important to continue to give your child their daily asthma medicine even if there are no visible symptoms of asthma. Long-term asthma medications can be left at home (if a child is at school or out of the house during the day) and are taken once or twice daily, depending on the medicine and the prescription.

53. Why are so many asthma medicines in inhaler form?

The inhaled route of delivering medication represents an ideal method for treating asthma. Asthma is a disease that involves the lungs and bronchial passageways. It therefore makes perfect sense to deliver the medicine directly where it is needed, right into the air passages. When it is inhaled, asthma medication goes precisely where it is required, with minimal, if any, absorption by other organs. By limiting the presence of medicine in the bloodstream and other organs, potential drug interactions are avoided and side effects and toxicity are minimized. Inhalers are practical, portable, and fit in a schoolbag, pocket, or handbag. They work at room temperature and can be taken without regard to meals or time of day. With proper instruction, motivated children as young as 5 or 6 years can be taught to successfully use inhaled medications, such as a metered-dose inhaler (MDI) or dry powder inhaler (DPI). The use of spacer devices such as holding chamber in combination with a metered-dose inhaler is recommended for children (and for adults who use the inhaler frequently) in order to maximize the effectiveness of their metered-dose inhalers.

54. How rapidly does medication delivered through an inhaler begin to work, and how long do the effects last?

The answer depends on which inhaler has been prescribed for your child. The medication's characteristics, rather than the method of delivery, determine its duration of action. Several different categories of inhaled asthma medicines exist, and each one has its own profile of action, so the answer to this question may vary depending on the type of inhaler and the specific medicine or type of inhaled medicine.

Inhaled asthma medications can generally be classified as either quick-relief or daily-use medicines. Quick-relief asthma

Dry powder inhaler (DPI)

A newer method of delivering medication directly to the lungs and respiratory passages. DPIs are supplanting traditional MDIs because of their ease of use, convenience, and good patient acceptance. Most children can learn to use DPIs effectively beginning at age 6 or above.

Treatment

medicines are designed to be used as needed, as soon as symptoms such as wheezing, breathlessness, or cough develop. Inhaled albuterol is an example of a quick-relief bronchodilator. When inhaled deeply and slowly, the medication begins to work right away—literally within minutes—to open up the constricted bronchial passages. The beneficial effects from a single dose (two puffs) can last for up to six hours.

Inhaled corticosteroid asthma medicines should be taken regularly whether or not symptoms are present. These medications are preventative in their action because they have the ability to decrease inflammation in the bronchial passageways and limit or block the development of asthma symptoms. The effectiveness of most maintenance asthma medicines increases during their first week of daily use; because they have a long duration of action, they are usually inhaled no more than once or twice a day at 12-hour intervals. For many patients, a single daily dose of their maintenance inhaled corticosteroid is all that is needed.

55. Why are some asthma medicines in metered-dose inhaler (MDI) form no longer manufactured?

Effective treatment of asthma requires the inhalation of bronchodilator and anti-inflammatory medicines. Metered-dose inhalers (MDIs) were first introduced in the 1950s. MDIs are used extensively in the treatment of asthma in both children and adults, and in other respiratory conditions such as emphysema and chronic obstructive bronchitis. Despite their complexity from an engineering perspective, MDIs are conceptually simple and user-friendly. They are small, convenient, and highly reliable devices that deliver precise doses of inhaled medication directly into the lungs' bronchial passageways. Many patients, and even some doctors, assume that MDIs are "all drug." In fact the traditional MDI also contains a propellant substance.

Until recently, all available MDIs used pharmaceutical grade chlorofluorocarbons (CFC) as propellants. Although CFCs are considered safe for individuals using MDIs, as they are chemically inert and do not accumulate in the body, they are harmful to the environment because they persist in the Earth's atmosphere for a long time and do damage to the Earth's ozone layer.

Ozone is a molecule made up of three oxygen atoms and is an essential constituent of our atmosphere. Approximately 90% of the ozone resides in a layer between six and twenty-five miles above the Earth's surface in a zone called the stratosphere. The presence of the correct amount of ozone in the Earth's stratosphere is crucial for absorbing dangerous radiation emanating from the sun. The stratosphere's ozone surrounds our planet in a protective envelope, in a sense. For example, increased exposure to the sun's ultraviolet rays, as would occur from depletion of the Earth's protective ozone layer, is associated with an increased risk for developing skin cancer and ocular cataracts in humans. Ozone depletion may also adversely affect animal and plant life.

The Montreal Protocol is a landmark, international treaty designed to enhance air quality and protect the uppermost (or stratospheric) ozone layer. In 1987, twenty-four countries and the European Economic Community negotiated and signed *The Montreal Protocol on Substances that Deplete the Ozone Layer*. The initial protocol had the goal of decreasing the use of ozone-depleting, man-made chemicals by 50% by the year 1999. Additional supplements to the Montreal Protocol, known as the London, Copenhagen, and Beijing Amendments, were adopted in 1990, 1992, and 1999, respectively, and further addressed the use and production of various ozone-depleting chemicals and provided a timetable for their phase-out.

Studies of the ozone layer over the last thirty years have shown a significant decline in the Earth's protective ozone

MDIs are small, convenient, and highly reliable devices that deliver precise doses of inhaled medication directly into the lungs' bronchial passageways.

Treatment

Chlorofluoro-carbons (CFCs)

Chemical propellants previously used in the manufacture of metered-dose inhalers. The manufacture and use of CFCs are now banned. A time-limited exception (due to expire in 2008) has been granted for certain inhalers until an equivalent replacement formulation is in production and available to patients.

layer over Antarctica. The first report of holes in the strato-spheric ozone layer by British scientists in May 1985 was subsequently confirmed and detailed. CFCs, which are widely used, have been implicated as a major source of atmospheric ozone depletion. CFCs contain chlorine, fluorine, and carbon atoms. CFCs were invented in the 1920s and are, in many ways, ideal compounds. CFCs are nontoxic, noncorrosive, and nonflammable. They are inert and nonreactive with most substances. In the second half of the twentieth century, CFCs were used extensively as propellants in aerosols and spray cans; as coolants in refrigerators and air conditioners; as solvents in cleaners, particularly for electronic circuit boards; and as blowing agents in the production of foam in devices such as fire extinguishers. Freon®, for example, is a familiar brand of a class of CFCs that was used in refrigeration. CFCs are chemically very stable, and experts now recognize that they can persist in the atmosphere for up to one hundred years. Therefore, even though the production and release of CFCs have been greatly curtailed, the damage to the ozone layer from past use will continue well into the current century.

The Montreal Protocol was codified by Congress into law in Title VI of the Clean Air Act and stipulated that the produc-tion of CFCs in consumer aerosols in the United States would be banned as of January 1, 1996. Existing medical products that contained CFCs were exempt from the ban until acceptable alternatives could be developed. An essential medical use of CFCs that is especially relevant to people with asthma is as a propellant in MDIs.

Although CFCs were no longer used in the manufacture of aerosol spray cans, air conditioners, or refrigeration units after January 1996, they were still produced for MDIs. Because MDIs are essential for asthma treatment, the Environmental Protection Agency (EPA) and the U.S. Food and Drug Admin-istration (FDA) extended the timeline banning CFC manu-facture, and proposed and oversaw the gradual phaseout of all MDIs containing CFCs (MDI-CFC). No CFC-containing

MDIs were removed from the market until a safe and effective equivalent medicine became available. A complete ban on the production and sale of single ingredient albuterol inhalers containing CFCs is scheduled to go into effect in the United States on December 31, 2008. The goal is to continue to develop CFC-free alternative MDIs and cease manufacture of CFCs. Several options in the marketplace now offer CFC-free alternatives.

Pharmaceutical manufacturers are either (1) reformulating their MDIs to be CFC-free or (2) developing inhaled drug-delivery systems that do not require any propellant at all. Reformulated albuterol MDIs substitute a different, non-CFC type of propellant called hydrofluoroalkane (HFA). The FDA has now approved three different CFC-free brands of albuterol sulfate bronchodilator MDIs, one brand of levalbuterol, one brand of MDI beclomethasone inhaled corticosteroid, and combinations of salmeterol combined with fluticasone and budesonide combined with panoterol that are all CFC-free. The products are Proventil® HFA, Ventolin® HFA, IVAX's albuterol MDI, Xopenex®, Qvar®, MDI Advair®, and MDI Symbicort®. Other CFC-free products are available in Europe, but are not currently approved by the FDA for use in the United States. In addition to producing HFA-propelled MDIs, pharmaceutical manufacturers have devised novel inhalers that do not rely on any propellant whatsoever. Several different controller asthma medicines are now available as dry powder inhalers (DPI) in the United States, and more are sure to follow.

Hydrofluoroalkane (HFA)

Medically inert substances that are used as propellants in metered-dose inhalers and meet chlorofluorocarbon-free criteria.

56. What do the letters "HFA" on my child's inhaler mean? Has the medicine been renamed?

Some parents have become concerned because of a change in the labeling of their child's metered-dose inhaler (MDI). All MDIs contain an active asthma medicine along with an inert material called a propellant. The propellant, as its name indicates, helps to propel the asthma medicine out of the canister into the lungs' breathing passages. The propellant is a substance called a hydrofluoroalkane, abbreviated HFA. As noted in Question 55, the propellant used in most MDIs until recently was a chlorofluorocarbon (CFC), which was found to play a key role in damaging the protective ozone layer of the atmosphere. At an international meeting held in Montréal, Canada in 1987, experts mandated that all CFC propellants should be replaced with a chemical that does not have the potential to destroy the ozone layer. HFA was the best choice to replace CFC. The reformulation of the propellant used in MDIs does not reduce the effectiveness of your child's inhaled medication. On the contrary, evidence suggests that the change from CFC to HFA propellant may, in the case of certain medicines, have actually increased the amount of medicine that is delivered "deeper" into the lung, reaching the smallest air passageways, a phenomenon that improves drug delivery in persons with asthma.

If, for example, your child is taking the Ventolin® HFA brand of albuterol manufactured by GlaxoSmithKline, you will notice that in addition to the trade name, Ventolin, the label also reads HFA. The active asthma medicine albuterol (a short-acting quick-relief β_2 agonist) in the newer HFA inhaler is identical to the albuterol in the older CFC inhaler; only the propellant is different. The medicine is the same and still carries the same name, and has the added benefit of including a dose counter and therefore more accurate because it specifies which inert propellant (HFA) is used in your child's MDI.

57. What is a Diskus®? Is it the same as a dry powder inhaler (DPI)?

The Diskus® is one of several types of dry powder inhaler (DPI) devices used in asthma treatment. Other devices that allow for inhalation of asthma medicines include the Turbuhaler®, the Diskhaler®, the Twisthaler®, and the Aerolizer®.

DPIs are devices that permit a person with asthma to self-administer precise, predetermined doses of inhaled corticosteroids or long-acting bronchodilators, either individually or in combination. DPIs were developed as an alternative delivery device to MDIs. From a technical point of view, patients usually find it easier to use a DPI than an MDI. It only requires that your child take a deep breath from the DPI mouthpiece for the medication, which is in the form of a very fine powder, to penetrate deeply into the bronchial passageways. Although DPIs and MDIs both dispense very precise doses of medication, DPIs are fundamentally different from MDIs. The DPI device automatically releases medicine as you generate an inward flow of air with your lips around the mouthpiece. The DPI is thus breath-activated or patient-activated. A child has to be able to generate sufficient airflow through the mouthpiece in order to benefit from a dry powder inhaler. As a general rule, DPIs are thus reserved for children over 5 years of age as younger children do not have the ability to generate the required airflow to trigger the release of medicine from the device.

Using an MDI, as compared to a DPI, requires a greater degree of coordination, timing, and skill to trigger the release the medicine just as you begin to inhale. You can expect that if your child is prescribed an MDI, the inhaler should be used with a dedicated spacer (or holding chamber) device. The younger the child, the more necessary it is for you to make certain that he or she use the MDI with a spacer device every time the medicine is needed, as detailed earlier in Table 21.

Some DPIs have a month's supply of asthma medicine already preloaded into the device. You bring up each dose as it is needed, usually by clicking a lever or twisting the base of the DPI unit immediately before use. Other DPIs require that you open the DPI before each inhalation and place a capsule that contains a single dose of medicine in powdered form into a groove before snapping the DPI back into place. Medicines provided through the Diskus®, Turbuhaler®, Clickhaler® and Twisthaler® are preloaded with a month's supply of medicine. The Aerolizer® requires that you to place a capsule containing

DPIs are devices that allow the self-administration of precisely measured doses of inhaled medicine.

the medicine into the device right before each use. The Dis-khaler® lets you load eight doses at once. The design of the Diskus® is distinctive and features a small counter that displays how many doses remain in the device, which is a very useful and practical feature.

Several different medicines come in DPI form, including long-acting β₂ agonists (such as salmeterol and formoterol), inhaled corticosteroids (such as budesonide, fluticasone, and mometasone), and combination DPIs containing different-potency inhaled corticosteroids, directly combined with long-acting β₂ agonists (such as mixtures of salmeterol and fluticasone). Trade names include the Serevent® Diskus, Foradil® Aerolizer, Pulmicort® Turbuhaler, Flovent® Diskus, Flovent® Rotadisk Diskhaler, Asmanex® Twisthaler, and Advair® Diskus.

58. What are corticosteroids (steroids), and how do they work?

Steroids are naturally occurring chemical substances (hormones) produced by the human body in health. The individual compounds that make up the steroid family have important roles in regulating many of the critical processes involved in our ability to function normally. Hormones are best described as chemical "messengers" produced in one organ and released into the bloodstream to exert their effects on another organ. The organs that produce steroids are the adrenal glands, the ovaries, and the testes. During pregnancy, an additional steroid-producing organ develops: the placenta, which produces the hormones required for the successful continuation of the pregnancy. The sex hormones estrogen and testosterone are synthesized by the ovary and testis, circulate in the bloodstream, and affect many different organs throughout the body. Similarly, the body's two adrenal glands produce adrenal cortical steroids (hydrocortisone, cortisone, aldosterone, and progesterone).

Scientists have succeeded in creating (or synthesizing) steroids in the laboratory for medical use. Corticosteroids have widespread usefulness in a diverse group of medical conditions. These steroid medicines are manufactured in different forms to treat a variety of specific conditions. You may be surprised to learn that corticosteroid medicines are manufactured as eye drops, nasal sprays, inhalers, creams and ointments, syrups, and pills, in an intravenous form, and even as a rectal suppository. Corticosteroids are invaluable to physicians who care for persons with inflammatory eye diseases such as uveitis, skin ailments such as psoriasis and eczema, rheumatologic diseases such as rheumatoid arthritis and lupus, inflammatory bowel diseases, some kidney diseases, and, of course, several lung diseases, especially asthma.

Corticosteroid medications are important because they have powerful anti-inflammatory effects; they reduce inflammation, which is the main problem in asthma and severe allergies. Corticosteroids in inhaled forms are the most effective asthma controller medicines available and are recommended asthma treatment for children of all ages. Inhaled corticosteroids are thus extensively used in asthma management.

59. My child was given a liquid cortisone medicine for a bad asthma attack. He had a very good response to this medicine. How does it work? Can he continue to take this medicine for a long time?

There are two major physiologic reactions that occur during an exacerbation of asthma. Initially, the muscles that surround the bronchi (air passageways) go into spasm (bronchospasm), which causes the airway to narrow (bronchoconstriction). The second and potentially more severe response involves several types of white blood cells: eosinophils, lymphocytes, mast cells, and neutrophils. When stimulated, these cells release a various chemicals called mediators, which cause the inflammatory reaction within the walls of the bronchial passageways. Physicians recognize that ongoing uncontrolled inflammation

Mediator

Chemical compounds that are either preformed or actively produced by specialized white blood cells as the result of an allergic reaction. These substances are responsible for the rapid onset of symptoms such as sneeze, runny nose, tearing eyes, cough, and wheeze, and the delayed development of inflammation.

Remodeling

Irreversible and permanent (anatomic and functional) changes that can occur in an asthmatic's lungs over time; thought to be a result of uncontrolled and untreated lung inflammation.

represents the greatest potential for producing chronic changes in your child's lungs. We now understand that this process can be a silent phenomenon, like high blood pressure or elevated cholesterol. A heightened inflammatory response is present to some degree in every child who has asthma, even in those with mild disease.

Asthma is now viewed as a chronic inflammatory disorder of the lungs. The response of the lungs to persistent inflammation may result in changes that never go away. These structural changes in the walls of the bronchial passageways can significantly alter the efficiency and effectiveness of your child's ability to breathe (see Question 19). The term currently used to describe this phenomenon is airway remodeling.

Traditionally, lung function abnormalities seen in bronchial asthma were considered a reversible phenomenon. Within the past two decades, our ideas about this concept have slowly been modified. There seems to be a subgroup of patients with asthma who appear to have greater degrees of inflammation in their lungs. Within this group, certain individuals' lung function never do return entirely to normal. It is unclear why exactly airway remodeling occurs. One hypothesis suggests that it results from unappreciated long-term effects of chronic asthmatic bronchial inflammation. However, the multiple factors responsible for the pathologic process called remodeling are still not completely understood.

Corticosteroids are effective in treating uncontrolled and persistent asthma because of their powerful anti-inflammatory properties. Today, these medications are unquestionably the preferred agents for the long-term treatment of anyone with persistent asthma symptoms. It must be emphasized that we are referring foremost to the administration of corticosteroid medications as inhaled aerosolized formulations delivered either through nebulizer, a dry powder inhaler, or a metered-dose inhaler, and not oral corticosteroids in either pill or liquid forms. It would be unusual today for a child with asthma to require the long-term use of oral steroids. In our own practices, for example, we have not found it necessary to start any child on a prolonged course of oral steroids in more than a decade! On the other hand, a short course (four to six days) of an oral steroid such as prednisone can effectively control an acute asthma exacerbation and is thus frequently used in clinical practice. Under these circumstances, the oral steroid is being used for a very limited time in order to "jump-start" the recovery process.

Whenever treatment with medications is being considered, and especially if corticosteroids are to be prescribed, the relative risks and benefits of these medications must be reviewed and discussed. Before inhaled formulations became available, the chronic use of oral (pill or liquid by mouth) corticosteroids was responsible both for saving many lives yet causing potentially life-threatening side effects. Because of the availability of inhaled (and nebulized) steroids, the potential for the development of serious systemic side effects has decreased dramatically. Of course, these drugs are pharmacologically potent. However, we do not hesitate to write a prescription for an inhaled steroid whenever the clinical situation is appropriate for either a child or an adult.

Obviously, no medication is entirely free of possible side effects. One question that often comes up relates to a possible effect of inhaled steroids on a child's growth. Note that uncontrolled asthma and severe asthma affect children's growth and will decrease final adult height. The most recent data shows that children with asthma who are treated with inhaled corticosteroids do ultimately reach their predicted adult height, but that it is reached at a later age. In particular, current evidence indicates that the rate of a child's growth may slow during the first year of inhaled steroid use. During the second year, most children who have experienced a decreased growth rate enter a catch-up growth phase. The accumulated data indicate that most of the time, children who have been using inhaled steroids for a long time reach their projected adult height.

It is very important to aggressively treat asthma symptoms whenever they appear.

Treatment

129

It is extremely important to understand that the long-term benefits associated with well-controlled asthma in virtually every case far outweigh the limited potential for developing harmful side effects associated with the proper use of inhaled steroids. It is a fact that poorly controlled asthma results in a long list of adverse side effects.

Other recognized possible side effects from inhaled steroid use include reversible throat irritation, hoarseness, and a localized yeast infection called *thrush*. Thrush occurs more commonly when inhaled corticosteroid particles "land" in the back of your child's throat. Measures that reduce the chances of contracting thrush include close attention to correct inhalation technique, using MDIs with a spacer device (such as a holding chamber), and rinsing the mouth and throat after inhaled steroid use. All patients who use inhaled corticosteroids, regardless of whether the medication is administered through metered-dose inhaler, dry powder inhaler, or by jet nebulizer, should rinse their mouth, gargle, and spit after each dose. The gargling and rinsing procedure will remove any residual steroid particles that may be trapped in the mouth or throat. If these steps are followed regularly after each dosing, the possibility of developing thrush or hoarseness will decrease dramatically.

It may be practical for your child to keep his or her inhaled MDI corticosteroid in the bathroom. They can then take their medication, brush their teeth, rinse their mouth, gargle, and spit. Since children brush their teeth twice a day, you can encourage the regular use of their controller medication by piggybacking the practice onto an already established habit pattern. Many children are agreeable to the suggestion. Note, however, that humid environments like bathrooms that become "steamed up" after showering are not good environments in which to store any of the dry powder inhalers (DPIs). The bathroom's high humidity can cause the DPI's fine medication particles to clump together and to lose their efficacy.

In summary, inhaled steroids are the preferred treatment for children who have been classified as having persistent asthma at any level of severity or who have any degree of uncontrolled asthma. Prednisone, as a liquid or tablet, should be used primarily as a quick-relief medication for relatively short periods (five to seven days) to control an acute exacerbation. The advantages of the inhaled corticosteroids unquestionably outweigh their potential side effects. Whenever your child is started on a treatment program that includes an inhaled steroid, he or she must be periodically reevaluated. As with any medication, the goal should always be to use the lowest dose of steroid possible to maintain your child in as near a normal state of function as possible. And finally, if your child is taking a steroid preparation and you have questions or concerns about the child's progress, do not hesitate to speak to either the asthma specialist or your primary care doctor. Remember, always attempt to get answers to your medical questions from a source as high up the information chain as possible.

It may be practical for your child to keep his or her inhaled MDI corticosteroid in the bathroom ... however, humid environments like bathrooms are not good environments in which to store dry powder inhalers (DPIs).

60. What are possible side effects of inhaled and oral steroids?

The potential side effects of steroids are well described in the medical literature and are related to (1) the route of administration, such as inhaled form (MDI, DPI, or nebulizer) or orally (pill or liquid), (2) the daily dose of steroid, (3) the total duration of steroid therapy, and (4) an individual variation in response to medication.

Inhaled corticosteroids have the best safety profile of all steroid preparations used to treat asthma. Inhaled corticosteroids are prescribed in one of three different forms: as a metered-dose inhaler (MDI), as a dry powder inhaler (DPI), or as a solution to be administered through a nebulizer. Inhaled corticosteroids are cornerstone asthma medications because they are the most effective anti-inflammatory treatment available. They are extremely useful controller medicines and help prevent asthma symptoms. Physicians who specialize in asthma

131

care generally prescribe an inhaled form of corticosteroid for maintenance or daily therapy and reserve oral (pill or liquid) steroids for treating an asthma flare or exacerbation. Possible side effects of inhaled corticosteroids include a hoarse voice, throat irritation, and thrush. Thrush is a mild yeast infection that occurs in the back of the throat and looks like small white blotches. Its treatment consists of an antifungal mouth rinse or occasionally a prescription for an antifungal pill. Using a spacer device with the MDI form of steroids, paying proper attention to careful inhalation technique, and gargling with water or a mouthwash after using the inhaler reduce the risk for developing any of these side effects as discussed above.

Inhaled corticosteroids have the best safety profile of all steroid preparations used to treat asthma.

Corticosteroids in pill, liquid, or injectable forms are called systemic steroids. Systemic means that the drug enters the blood circulation and is distributed throughout the body (systemically). The steroids enter the lung circulation, where they exert tremendous beneficial effects in exacerbated asthma, but they also penetrate into other organs, such as the skin, eyes, brain, and bone. Because systemic corticosteroids circulate in higher concentrations throughout the body, they (1) have a greater potential than inhaled corticosteroids to cause side effects, and (2) can, especially with prolonged use, lead to multiple adverse effects involving many organ systems. A person who requires 60 mg of prednisone daily for six weeks, for example (an admittedly unusually high and prolonged dose in asthma treatment, but not unheard of in the treatment of certain serious illnesses), can expect to develop more significant side effects compared with a person taking 40 mg of prednisone for one day, 35 mg the next day, then 30 mg the day after, and so forth, tapering down by 5 mg each day for a total of eight days of therapy.

Because everyone is unique in how they respond to medications, steroids can affect people in different ways. Oral steroids are used only for brief periods (on the order of days) in the treatment of childhood asthma to gain control of an exacerbation. Oral steroids' rapid onset of beneficial action in the treatment of uncontrolled asthma means that if your child is prescribed prednisone or methylprednisolone, for example, the treatment course will be short. It is thus very unlikely that your child will remain on the oral steroid long enough to develop the side effects that can be seen with long-term steroid usage. But what exactly can be the potential side effects of longer term oral steroid treatment? We know the possible answers from studies of steroids used in medical conditions other than asthma. Such conditions include illnesses such as inflammatory bowel disease, systemic lupus, certain kinds of kidney diseases, as well as examples from the fields of transplant medicine, hematology and oncology. In general, systemic steroids cause mood elevation and increased energy in adults, but children sometimes get depressed while taking them. Some children may experience insomnia. Steroids stimulate appetite and food tastes better. Because steroids can cause water retention and increased appetite, weight gain may occur, particularly with longer duration of use. In adults more than in children, steroids can cause blood pressure to rise and can cause glucose intolerance, which makes preexisting diabetes harder to control. Oral steroids taken chronically may affect the rate of a child's growth. Bone weakness and elevations in the pressure of the eye have also been described in children who need high doses of steroids orally for months at a time. With long-term use, steroids can lead to acne and cause the skin to bruise easily. Some people develop a rounded facial appearance (moon face) that, like many other steroid side effects, is not permanent and disappears after the steroid medication has been tapered and discontinued.

Significant systemic side effects are extremely unusual with inhaled corticosteroids. The serious adverse effects of corticosteroids occur with long-term, chronic oral steroid use, ranging from many months to years, and are seldom seen with contemporary asthma treatment. It is unusual to encounter significant side effects, even in children requiring a 5- to 7-day burst of systemic steroids to treat a flare of asthma symptoms, for example. Remember that when an asthma exacerbation is identified early

Glucose intolerance

A condition in which the body shows some degree of resistance to insulin, so it can't move glucose into cells efficiently and utilize it as an efficient body fuel. This condition can range from "prediabetes," in which high blood glucose is notably above normal after a fast but below levels diagnostic of diabetes, to Type 2 diabetes.

and treated promptly, the intensity and length of corticosteroid quick-relief medication required to control the episode will be much less than if the flare-up of symptoms is allowed to progress to where hospitalization is necessary. Asthma experts believe that optimal treatment of worsening asthma symptoms is paramount, and that any theoretical concerns you may harbor about the remote possibility of significant side effects should never interfere with the decision to use corticosteroids in asthma treatment.

61. Are corticosteroids dangerous?

No, not if your child takes the steroids exactly as prescribed. Every prescription medication sold in the United States has passed the U.S. Food and Drug Administration's rigorous approval process. Corticosteroids are no exception; like any other class of medicine, steroids are safe and effective when prescribed appropriately and when used exactly as directed. Steroids are not inherently any more or less dangerous than other medicines. Like any other medicine, they have potential side effects, especially if used in pill form chronically (long-term) and in large doses.

Anabolic steroids

Compounds normally produced by the body in health that have the capacity to increase muscle mass, among other effects. Anabolic steroids are unrelated to the corticosteroids used in asthma treatment but are sometimes confused with such medications because of the common use of "steroids" to refer to both types of compounds.

Steroid preparations have important and diverse medical uses. The development of inhaled corticosteroid medicines in metered-dose inhaler, nebulized, and dry powder inhaler forms has revolutionized the treatment of asthma and positively transformed the lives of countless people with asthma. Steroids come in forms other than pills and inhalers. An allergic child with eczema may be treated with a steroid cream, for example. Similarly, ophthalmologists may prescribe steroid eye drops for specific conditions. Steroids are a powerful medicine in the allergist's and pulmonologist's armamentarium, and can be lifesaving in certain medical situations, such as a severe exacerbation of asthma.

Why, then, might people think of steroids as dangerous? Some confuse anabolic steroids with corticosteroids. Anabolic steroids have been abused by some weight builders and athletes to help them bulk up and build muscle mass, and they have a reputation for causing dangerous side effects when misused. Corticosteroids are completely different medicines than anabolic steroids, and are the class of steroid medication used extensively in treatment of allergy and asthma. The only "danger" to using them occurs if they are not used correctly. It is critically important to follow the dosing schedule exactly as outlined by your child's physician. If your child requires daily oral steroids, it is vitally important that you follow the physician's dosing recommendations. A child who is has been prescribed daily oral corticosteroid treatment has moderate to severe persistent asthma and requires the corticosteroid for asthma control. You will unnecessarily place your child in danger if you (1) fail to stay in close contact with the treating physician regarding your child's clinical condition and (2) if you deviate in any way from the previously established oral steroid dosing schedule without first discussing the situation with the physician. There are in particular at least two important reasons why an asthma patient should not abruptly stop taking the pill form of corticosteroids. The first reason is that since the steroids are prescribed for asthma treatment, there is a good chance that the asthma will flare anew if the steroid dosage is decreased too rapidly or all at once. The second reason applies to individuals who require steroids on a more long-term basis as discussed next.

Our bodies produce a natural form of steroids that is required for health. The adrenal glands located above each kidney are responsible for meeting the body's corticosteroid requirements. The steroids produced by the adrenal glands are referred to as the body's endogenous steroids. When the adrenal glands detect extra steroids in the bloodstream from medication, they reduce their own endogenous steroid production. If the adrenal glands are exposed to a significant amount of steroid medication, they respond by completely shutting down the body's own vital manufacture of steroids.

Endogenous steroids

Steroids normally produced in health by the body's adrenal glands.

When people continue to take their prescribed steroid medication, the adrenals remain "sluggish and turned off" and stop producing endogenous steroids. When steroid medication is reduced gradually, the adrenal glands have time to respond and resume producing enough endogenous steroids to meet the body's needs. If, on the other hand, long-term steroid pills are not tapered and are stopped abruptly, the adrenal glands will not have sufficient time to recover and restart manufacturing endogenous steroids. The body will be left without any steroids at all, and an adrenal crisis, which is a true medical emergency, may ensue. The treatment of adrenal crisis includes steroid administration.

When your child's asthma becomes controlled and it becomes medically appropriate to discontinue oral steroid treatment, your physician will provide you with a detailed dosage schedule that will slowly decrease or "taper off" the use of the medication. This will permit the adrenal glands to "awaken" and once again begin to produce essential ndogenous steroids. The most critical point is to work closely with the physician and avoid making decisions regarding these medications without appropriate consultation.

Steroids are considered safe when taken exactly as prescribed for appropriate medical indications. Let's say that your teenage daughter's asthma has become more active and is becoming uncontrolled. Despite the fact that she is using daily inhaled, long-acting β_2 agonists along with an inhaled, high-dose corticosteroid, she also now requires a short-acting quick-relief inhaled β_2 agonist every four to six hours for relief of breathlessness. Her peak flow measurements have decreased. She is also awakening at night because of respiratory difficulty. She tells you that she is feeling "rotten." At this point, her physician will undoubtedly recommend a course of oral steroids (steroid burst). When dealing with children, a short course (pulse or burst dose) of oral prednisone is usually prescribed for five to seven days. In older teenagers or adults, the steroid burst may be continued for a somewhat longer period.

When the duration of treatment is seven days or less, there is generally no need to taper the prednisone dose. However, for steroid treatment extending over a longer period, there should be a gradual daily decrease (taper) of the dose. Your daughter can expect to experience an improvement in her asthma exacerbation, with lessening of symptoms in as little as six to twelve hours after the first dose of steroids.

When used properly, steroids can be almost miraculous in their effectiveness. Prednisone and methylprednisolone are two different steroids in pill or liquid (oral) form that are frequently prescribed to treat asthma exacerbations and severe allergic reactions. The NAEEP guidelines point out that prednisone or methylprednisolone may sometimes be required in small daily doses to treat severe persistent asthma. A 5-mg dose of prednisone is equivalent to a 4-mg dose of methylprednisolone. We usually advise our patients who require steroids to start taking them early and get off them as quickly as possible so that they can take advantage of the beneficial qualities when treating an exacerbation and minimize potential side effects. Also note that if you believe your child's asthma requires treatment with an oral steroid, you must urgently contact the child's physician. We firmly believe that adding oral corticosteroid medicine to your child's asthma regimen unquestionably requires a conversation between you and your child's physician to provide your child with the most appropriate treatment recommendations.

Steroids are considered safe when taken exactly as prescribed for appropriate medical indications.

Kerrin's comment:

My son was prescribed Pulmicort® Respules® after being hospitalized for respiratory problems. We've been instructed to use it in the nebulizer after the albuterol (which we were told opens up the breathing passages to then allow the steroid better movement) whenever we believe his breathing is becoming compromised. It's a steroid, but it has helped keep him out of the hospital (where he would receive steroids anyway) several times, so whatever the possible side effects, they're worth it.

62. How do asthma medicines work (such as theophylline, albuterol, levalbuterol, montelukast, inhaled corticosteroids, fluticasone/salmeterol)?

Theophylline, albuterol, levalbuterol, formoterol, and salmeterol are all bronchodilators; they work by opening constricted bronchial passages. Albuterol, levalbuterol, formoterol, and salmeterol exert their beneficial respiratory effects by stimulating the lungs' β_2 receptors. Doctors refer to them as beta agonists (β_2 agonists). Human lungs have specialized microscopic receptors called β_2 receptors. When a β_2 agonist medicine attaches to the lung's β_2 receptors through chemical binding and stimulates the β_2 receptor, the muscles surrounding the bronchial tubes relax (bronchodilate) and allow for an easier flow of air. Inhaled albuterol and levalbuterol are short-acting β_2 quick-relief bronchodilators in asthma treatment plans. Their onset of action is rapid, occurring within minutes. On the other end of the spectrum, salmeterol and formoterol are considered long-acting β_2 agonists and have a longer duration of action, lasting up to twelve hours as compared with albuterol or levalbuterol, which only last about six hours. The long-acting β_2 agonists (salmeterol and formoterol) are usually considered to be daily-use long-term control bronchodilators in asthma management.

Theophylline, although a bronchodilator, does not attach to the lungs' β_2 receptors, so it is not a β_2 agonist or stimulant. It acts through a completely separate chemical pathway. Theophylline, unlike the β_2 agonist medicines, is not manufactured in an inhaled form. Theophylline is not used as a first-line treatment in contemporary asthma management. Theophylline is available as a pill, capsule, or liquid elixir and must be taken every twelve hours. Many other oral medications, including antibiotics, can affect how the body metabolizes theophylline. If your child takes theophylline as a maintenance asthma treatment, always check with the physician when your child is started on a new medicine. It is important to ensure that no potential undesirable drug interaction occur between the the-ophylline and the new medicine. A reduction in theophylline dosage may sometimes be required. Theophylline, along with salmeterol, formoterol, montelukast, and the inhaled cortico-steroids, is classified as a daily-use control medication.

Montelukast is an oral asthma medication that also exhib-its antiallergy properties. Montelukast is a daily-use control medicine that is approved by the U.S. Food and Drug Ad-ministration for treating mild intermittent and mild persistent asthma, exercise-induced bronchoconstriction, and allergic rhinitis. Montelukast may be a good choice for children with very mild forms of asthma who also have nasal allergies and is approved for use in children as young as 2 years of age. In older kids and adults, it seems to be effective in treat-ing exercise-induced asthma. It works by preventing certain inflammatory proteins called leukotrienes from attaching to specialized receptors on cells. By blocking the attachment of leukotrienes, montelukast controls asthmatic inflammation. Doctors refer to montelukast as a leukotriene antagonist or a leukotriene modifier and consider it a daily maintenance, controller asthma therapy. There are currently three leukot-riene modifiers on the American market: montelukast for patients 2 years and older, zafirlukast for patients 5 and older, and zileuton for ages 12 and up.

There are six different inhaled corticosteroid medications on the U.S. market that differ slightly from one another in their potency and delivery systems (metered-dose inhaler vs. dry powder inhaler vs. nebulizer). All inhaled corticosteroid agents share a common mechanism of action. The currently available inhaled corticosteroids on the market in the United States include flunisolide, mometasone, triamcinolone, fluticasone, budesonide, and beclomethasone. Nebulized budesonide is FDA approved for children as young as a year of age, and DPI fluticasone is approved for children beginning at the age of 4 years. All inhaled corticosteroids are daily-use long-term con-trol maintenance medicines that reduce lung inflammation and potentially prevent asthma symptoms, attacks, and exacerbations. Inhaled corticosteroids are not bronchodilators and are consequently ineffective in rapidly reversing narrowing of the bronchial tubes (bronchoconstriction). They should be taken as prescribed, on a routine, daily basis, and are often prescribed with an inhaled bronchodilator such as albuterol, levalbuterol, or salmeterol. Most specialists advise that your child rinse his or her mouth and throat with tap water or mouthwash after inhaling any corticosteroid medicines (see Question 59).

Fluticasone and salmeterol are two maintenance medicines that are especially effective when used together in the long-term treatment of asthma. Their mechanisms of action complement one another. Fluticasone, an inhaled steroid, is anti-inflammatory in its action, and salmeterol is a long-acting bronchodilator. They work together to control the two pathologic processes present in asthma: inflammation and bronchoconstriction. The trade name for the combination of fluticasone and salmeterol is Advair®. Advair® is manufactured as both a metered-dose inhaler (MDI) and as a dry powder inhaler called a Diskus®. Only the latter is FDA approved for use in children as of this writing; Advair® in MDI form is reserved for patients ages 18 years and above. Advair® used in the treatment of asthma in children and young teens is manufactured in three strengths in depending on the concentration of fluticasone, the inhaled corticosteroid. Advair®Diskus is currently available in the following strengths: 100/50, 250/50, and 500/50. The recommended regimen is one inhalation twice a day, approximately twelve hours apart. After each dose, children should rinse their mouth with water, gargle, and then spit. This action will remove any steroid particles that may have become trapped in the throat area. The lowest dosage, 100/50, is recommended for children ages 4 to 11 years. Each puff of Advair® regardless of its strength contains an identical dose of the long-acting β_2 bronchodilator, salmeterol (50 mcg). The difference between the three dosage forms relates to the amount of the steroid, fluticasone, which ranges from 100 mcg to 250 mcg and finally 500 mcg in each inhalation. A practical consequence of the fixed combination of medicines contained in Advair® is that the dose should never be increased beyond the one puff twice a day. Taking extra puffs of Advair® in excess of what the physician has instructed may lead to an overdose of the salmeterol component, which can be very serious and potentially harmful.

63. How do the different medicines my son uses actually work? Is it necessary for him to carry his "puffer" all the time?

The device that many patients and their parents sometimes refer to as a puffer is technically a pressurized metered-dose inhaler (MDI). Every time a MDI is activated, a premeasured dose of medicine is released. The aerosolized medication must be inhaled slowly and deeply into the bronchial passageways for it to be most effective. Once the technical aspects of using an MDI have been mastered, it becomes a highly effective delivery system for various anti-asthma medicines.

Most children with asthma currently use an inhaler that contains a short-acting bronchodilator, typically albuterol. Albuterol belongs to the class of anti-asthma drugs termed fast-acting, rapid-response, quick-relief medications. All children who have asthma, with few exceptions, should have their quick-relief medication with them or close by at all times.

All children who have asthma, with few exceptions, should have their quick-relief medication with them or close by at all times.

Many different medicines are available for treating childhood asthma and are divided into two main groups based on their role in asthma treatment. They are either daily control medicines (for long-term maintenance) or fast-acting (for providing quick relief) medications (Table 22). Controller medications should be taken daily, whereas the fast-acting or reliever drugs are used when a child experiences a sudden flare or exacerbation of asthma symptoms. Controller maintenance medications (such as inhaled corticosteroids, or oral montelukast) must be taken regularly once or twice a day depending on the medication. Your child obviously does not need to keep his prescribed long-term control medicine on his person at all times and can thus keep it at home. However, because you never know when a situation may arise that might precipitate the sudden onset of asthma symptoms, your child should always carry his fast-acting medicine (such as albuterol) with him at all times just in case.

Table 22   Asthma Medications: Effects on Asthma

Reliever/Quick-Relief Medications:	
Short-acting bronchodilators	Rapidly relieve bronchial constriction, decreasing cough and wheeze
Anticholinergic agents	Affect the portion of the nervous system (cholinergic nerves) that contributes to cough and mucus production
"Burst" oral corticosteroids	Potent anti-inflammatory agents that decrease inflammation, swelling, and irritation of the bronchial passageways

Controller /Maintenance Medications are used daily and include:	
Inhaled corticosteroids	Decrease or block inflammation
Long-acting bronchodilators	Relieve bronchoconstriction by relaxing the muscle spasm that causes narrowing of the bronchial passageways
Mast cell stabilizers	Block the release of mediators from the mast cell, minimizing the development of symptoms
Leukotriene receptor antagonists	Block the attachment of leukotrienes to target cells, thereby minimizing inflammation and improving long-term control.

Medications in the daily use maintenance category include inhaled corticosteroids, long-acting bronchodilators, mast cell stabilizers, and anti-leukotriene receptor antagonists. These various drugs have different mechanisms of action (Table 22).

They ultimately decrease (or possibly eliminate) inflammation, thereby minimizing and preventing the development of clinical asthma symptoms. Inhaled corticosteroids decrease or block inflammation, whereas long-acting bronchodilators relieve bronchoconstriction by relaxing the muscle spasm that causes narrowing of the bronchial passageways.

The mast cell (a member of the white blood cell family) plays a major role in allergic reactions. When the mast cell is stimulated, it releases many chemical substances (mediators) that are responsible for causing asthma symptoms, such as cough and wheeze. The mast cell stabilizers can block the release of mediators from the mast cell, thereby curtailing the development of symptoms.

The leukotrienes are different chemical mediators that play a role in the development of the inflammatory response in asthma. By either interfering with the production of leukotrienes or by preventing leukotrienes from attaching to specialized leukotriene receptors on lung cells, the leukotriene receptor antagonist group of medicines minimize inflammation and thereby improve the long-term outcome for your child's asthma.

Asthma medicines of the fast-acting or quick-relief class consist of short-acting bronchodilators, short (pulse or burst) courses of oral steroids (five to seven days), and anticholinergic drugs. All are used to relieve acute symptoms, such as cough, tightness, and wheeze. Short-acting quick-relief bronchodilators begin to work rapidly to relieve muscle spasm, which in turn helps to decrease cough and wheeze. A single dose (two puffs of the rapid-acting quick-relief MDI) usually provides symptom control for two to six hours. Anticholinergic agents affect the portion of the nervous system (cholinergic nerves) that is responsible for triggering a cough. Their primary effectiveness is in controlling cough. These agents are often combined in a single MDI with a short-acting bronchodilator. An example of such a combination is Combivent®, which is a

Treatment

combination of ipratropium and albuterol in one MDI. One dose is effective for two to six hours, and it is usually taken every four to six hours.

Oral corticosteroids are potent anti-inflammatory agents that decrease inflammation, swelling, and irritation of the bronchial passageways. Oral steroids are usually prescribed in one of two clinical circumstances. First, they are used as a quick-relief treatment, prescribed as a "burst" for less than a week to control the acute onset of severe symptoms. The use of the oral steroid agent combined with a short-acting bronchodilator is generally effective in controlling acute symptoms. Secondly, daily oral corticosteroids are used to treat the relatively rare and unusual patient whose asthma symptoms remain uncontrolled or poorly controlled despite adherence to a comprehensive anti-asthma drug program. Such a child would be started on a long-term, low-dose oral daily steroid regimen in addition to the other medicines that were prescribed. Step 6 asthma treatment outlined in the latest NAEPP guidelines includes patients who require oral corticosteroids as daily asthma treatment. Those children must be under the continued care of a medical specialist in asthma care.

64. Is it necessary to take asthma medicine every day? When my daughter stops coughing and wheezing, can she stop taking the medicine? Is it necessary for her to use all three medicines the doctor prescribed?

The answer is definitely yes, if that is what your daughter's physician has prescribed. A great advance in understanding asthma is the recognition that inflammation within the bronchial passageways is the crucial factor in the pathophysiology of the disease. If a child with asthma has persistent inflammation involving her lungs, it will be close to impossible to properly control her symptoms. Too many children with inadequately treated asthma limit or change their daily activities and thereby learn to "live with their disease." The correct approach to this situation is not to "give in" to the problem but rather to get proper treatment so that you control the disease rather than the other way around.

The primary treatment goals for asthma control include the absence of symptoms day and night. If your child's asthma is causing symptoms three or more times a week it is considered to be out of control. Treatment under these cirumstances should include a quick-relief bronchodilator and a daily-use maintence anti-inflamatory medication. As outlined in the asthma guidelines published by the National Asthma Education and Prevention Program (NAEPP) and by the Global Initiative for Asthma (GINA), primary treatment goals include the absence of daily daytime and nighttime symptoms. Breathing should always be comfortable. Cough and wheeze should be absent. If your child's asthma falls into a classification other than controlled in the GINA guidelines and mild intermittent according to the NAEPP guidelines, then she should be treated with a daily controller medication and a quick-relief, or fast-acting, MDI.

Asthma medicine can be classified into two broad categories: as-needed rapid acting quick-relief treatments and long-term maintenance control daily-use treatments (see Question 52). Those children with mild intermittent asthma only use their medicine when they are actively symptomatic. They do not require any pre-programmed daily medicine. Others with more pronounced asthma must, however, take maintenance controller medicine every day even though they are free of symptoms and feel perfectly well.

Long-term daily use of inhaled medicines address the inflammatory component of asthma. The medicines are designed to be taken every day to diminish and control inflammation. They are preventive maintenance medicines. Your child should use them as prescribed, whether or not obvious symptoms are present. The fact that your child has no symptoms means that the medicine is working effectively and that she should continue taking it. If your child stops taking the medicine because she feels fine, she may not feel fine for long. Rather than allow your child to stop taking the medicine, you should discuss the situation with her physician. The fact that she feels healthy certainly indicates that her treatment has been effective. It may also indicate that your child may be ready to decrease, or step down, that particular treatment. Experts advise that, as a rule, asthma be well controlled for three months (90 consecutive days) and that lung function tests be within a normal (or close to normal) range before proceeding with a step down in asthma medication.

65. Do children with asthma have to take their medicine all year-round?

Some do, and some do not. Asthma is a variable disease, both from person to person and over time for a particular child. Several circumstances will determine how the question is answered for an individual child. Treatment recommendations vary depending on the severity and frequency of your child's symptoms, the degree of control obtained with treatment, and the ease with which that control is obtained. If cough and wheeze occur infrequently, your child has intermittent asthma. If these symptoms are present more than twice a week, then your child has persistent asthma according to the current NAEPP classification. Persistent asthma is further subdivided into mild, moderate, and severe categories. Regardless of symptom level, any child with asthma, even one with a mild classification at time of diagnosis, may experience a severe attack at any time; this point cannot be stressed too strongly. The NAEPP provides clinicians with a schema of a stepwise approach to asthma treatment, with six steps based on an individual child's symptoms, night-time awakenings, need for short-acting β_2 inhaled bronchodilators, and for children 5 years and older, assessment of lung function. The concept is that an individual child should have appropriate therapy at the onset and then periodic reassessments as time passes to determine how effective the asthma treatment is.

A "step down" in the intensity of pharmacologic treatment is appropriate when your child's asthma has responded well and is controlled and asymptomatic, and a "step up" must be prescribed when, on the other hand, a child continues to experience asthma symptoms and their disease is not controlled.

Children with milder asthma may only need to use a short-acting bronchodilator, such as albuterol, when they are symptomatic. The medication should be given every four to six hours beginning with the earliest signs and symptoms of cough, wheeze, or chest tightness and continued until your child has been symptom-free for at least four or five days. If the symptoms do not improve within the first twenty-four to thirty-six hours, a controller medication such as an inhaled corticosteroid may be started. The inhaled corticosteroid preparation should be continued for at least ten to fourteen days after the symptoms have cleared. It is always best to speak with the doctor and make certain you understand about when to stop or decrease (step down) any medication that has been prescribed for your child.

Treatment recommendations vary depending on the severity and frequency of symptoms, the degree of control achieved with treatment, and the ease with which control is obtained.

The recommendations are different if your child has persistent or poorly controlled asthma of any severity. A daily controller medication, preferably an inhaled corticosteroid, or possibly a combined preparation containing a corticosteroid and a long-acting bronchodilator (fluticasone plus salmeterol) or a nonsteroid anti-leukotriene receptor antagonist (montelukast), should be taken every day. The recommendation is based on the knowledge that inflammation is an ongoing process occurring in poorly controlled or persistent asthma. Although a definitive statement cannot yet be made, experts are cautiously optimistic that this approach will improve the long-term prognosis and lead to normal or near-normal lung function in children who have persistent asthma. Ongoing studies are looking at various treatment options in order to provide specific answers about the long-term outcome for these children.

147

As parents and involved physicians, we can appreciate the frequently asked question, "when is it safe to stop giving my child medicine?" Unfortunately, not enough information is available to give an absolute answer, and the answer to this question would depend on individual circumstances in any case. Our current recommendation for the continued use of maintenance controller asthma medications would be to discuss the situation with your child's physicians and take no action unless everyone agrees what is best for your child.

66. Why is it important for my child to use a medicine such as albuterol when he wheezes or coughs, and an inhaled corticosteroid medicine when he seems to be free of his symptoms?

Your very important question provides the opportunity to review basic concepts about our current understanding of the pathophysiology of bronchial asthma. Nancy Sander, the founder and president of a national asthma patient advocacy organization called "Mothers of Asthmatics," recently talked about "the asthma you see" and "the asthma you don't see."

The "asthma you see" refers to the obvious symptoms of cough, wheeze, shortness of breath, and complaints of difficulty breathing that asthma patients experience. More than forty years ago, allergists and chest specialists felt as though they had accomplished something significant when they succeeded in stopping a child from coughing or wheezing. The main treatment goal then for asthma patients was to control the chest symptoms characteristic of asthma. At that time, physicians did not understand the potential adverse outcomes associated with "the asthma you don't see" related to the effects of bronchial inflammation. During the past fifteen to twenty years, we have come to appreciate the significant role bronchial inflammation plays in virtually all patients who have this disease. Today, it is critically important for your child's asthma health care team to not only focus on relieving the obvious symptoms of asthma but also to control the potentially more harmful effects of unsuspected inflammation. Ongoing lung inflammation can be a silent process, causing significant pathologic changes within the lungs that may result in irreversible pulmonary damage.

To answer the original question, albuterol falls into the class of asthma medicines currently described as relievers or fast-relief drugs. For example, if a child who has asthma began to cough or wheeze, he should use either albuterol (Proventil® HFA or Ventolin® HFA) or levalbuterol (Xopenex® HFA), or pirbuterol (Maxair®) to rapidly relieve his symptoms of cough and wheeze.

Medications used to address the underlying ("invisible") inflammation of asthma include inhaled corticosteroid preparations and leukotriene receptor antagonists. Anti-inflammatory medicines should thus be taken in addition to any quick-relief, fast-acting bronchodilator inhalers needed to treat "the asthma you see." Inhaled corticosteroids and leukotriene receptor antagonists are prescribed for daily use and must be taken regularly, for weeks, months, and, in some cases, years. The medicines are prescribed to control the harmful long-term effects of increased lung inflammation. The reason for taking them on a long-term basis reflects increasing knowledge about the chronic nature of lung inflammation in asthma and the potential anatomic changes that can occur from this persistent process when it is not adequately treated. Over time, irreversible physical changes may occur within the lungs, a phenomenon known as airway remodeling (see Question 19).

Advances in the understanding of asthma explains why your child's doctor will prescribe some medicines to be taken on an as-needed schedule (fast-acting quick relievers) and others (anti-inflammatory maintenance controllers) on a daily schedule for an extended period as an important part of a maintenance program.

Treatment

67. What is exercise-induced asthma? How is it different from exercise-induced bronchospasm?

Exercise is a universal and common asthma trigger. Individuals with inadequately controlled asthma often experience variable cough, wheezing, and breathlessness with exertion and aerobic exercise. The reversible airway narrowing that occurs during and (more commonly) after exercise is called exercise-induced bronchospasm (EIB). Anyone with asthma is at risk for EIB, but up to 10% of persons who experience EIB are neither atopic nor asthmatic. Nonasthmatic persons with EIB are often very athletic and are believed to have a separate condition called exercise-induced asthma, or EIA. Controversy and misunderstanding surround this terminology, which attempts to describe a clinical phenomenon (bronchoconstriction) in the absence of an asthma diagnosis. Adding to the confusion, some physicians consider EIA as a subtype of asthma, although others view it as a possible precursor to asthma. We prefer to use the admittedly wordy but descriptive terms "exercise-induced bronchospasm in the setting of underlying asthma" and "exercise-induced bronchospasm without asthma" for maximal clarity. In the first scenario, exercise is a typical trigger among others for asthma, whereas in the second, exercise is the sole stimulus of cough, wheezing, chest tightness, and dyspnea.

What do we know about the EIB that occurs in the absence of underlying asthma and atopy, a phenomenon also named EIA? Studies in athletes show that up to one-quarter of Olympic winter sports athletes experience EIB. The numbers are highest (50%) in cross-country skiers. The U.S. Olympic Committee found that 11.2% of athletes competing in the 1984 Summer Olympics experienced EIB. Remember that EIB without asthma, often (confusingly) called EIA, is a clinically different phenomenon from EIB with asthma and cannot (by definition) reflect inadequately controlled asthma. Individuals with exercise-induced bronchospasm (who are "not asthmatic")

Atopy/Atopic

Atopy is an inherited predisposition to the development of allergic conditions such as hay fever, eczema, allergic rhinitis, and even certain forms of asthma. A person with evidence of atopy is said to be atopic.

experience respiratory symptoms only in the setting of aerobic exercise. The symptoms may include dry cough, wheezing, and shortness of breath, along with chest discomfort. The symptoms can begin as early as a few minutes after beginning exercise and typically increase after exercise ends, usually peaking five to ten minutes after maximal exercise ceases. Symptoms can continue to peak for another thirty minutes after sports, although some athletes experience EIB symptoms for more extended periods. Decreased performance usually ensues.

Treatment includes proper attention to warm-up and cool-down maneuvers and prescription medication. Medicines effective in treating EIB/EIA include oral leukotriene modifiers and inhaled short-acting β_2 agonists, inhaled long-acting β_2 agonists, and/or inhaled cromolyn. Several different medications can be prescribed if required. If inhalers are prescribed, they should be used approximately twenty minutes before the warm-up routine. In EIA, airway narrowing occurs secondary to vigorous exercise. The mechanism responsible for EIA implicates inhalation of cold dry air, specifically changes in humidity and temperature within the airways during rapid breathing.

68. Whenever my daughter plays soccer, she begins to cough and she sometimes says that her chest feels "tight." Could this be some form of asthma? Will she need to stop participating in sports?

Complaints of cough, wheeze, chest pain, feelings of chest tightness, or shortness of breath that occur during strenuous physical exertion are symptoms suggestive of exercise-induced bronchospasm (EIB). For many children, such symptoms be the first indication that they have asthma. A very high percentage of patients with asthma will at some time have respiratory symptoms triggered by vigorous exercise.

Complaints of cough, wheeze, chest pain, a sensation of chest tightness, or shortness of breath that occur during strenuous physical exertion are symptoms consistent with a diagnosis of exercise-induced bronchospasm.

During periods of intense physical activity, children not only breathe more rapidly, but also breathe through their mouths rather than through their noses. A major physiologic function of the nose is to filter, humidify, and warm the air before it reaches the lungs. So, during active participation in sports, since we preferentially breathe through our mouth rather than the nose, the air that enters the lungs is unfiltered, cold, and dry.

Although we do not have a complete understanding of the exact mechanisms of EIB, experts believe that chest symptoms develop because of the rapid intake of large volumes of cold, dry air. As an analogy, consider two weather fronts coming together with a disturbance developing at the point where they collide. For example, John is a 6-year-old soccer player who, as he begins to run up and down the soccer field on a cool, some-what windy day in late October, suddenly begins to cough and his chest feels tight. In this example, John develops symptoms because he is sucking in large amounts of relatively cold, late October air. When this air mass reaches his upper airway, a reaction is triggered that causes his symptoms to develop. This is a common initial presentation of a child who has EIB.

Fortunately most children who have EIB do not have to limit their physical activities. Years ago, asthma specialists suggested that children with asthma should limit or stop their participation in gym class and team sports. At that time, it was falsely believed that limited activity was best for children who had asthma. Today, because so much more is understood about the disease, combined with the availability of more effective medications, children with asthma should be able to enjoy a full, active athletic life. Regular aerobic exercise is, in fact, part of a successful asthma treatment program!

Several medications are currently used to treat EIB. The treating physician will recommend which one is best for your child. The possibilities include: inhaled short-acting β_2 agonists (albuterol), inhaled long-acting β_2 agonists (salmeterol), inhaled mast cell stabilizers (cromolyn), and oral leukotriene modifiers (montelukast). Several different medications can be prescribed if required. Of the several medications, albuterol has been very effective for most patients with exercise-induced bronchospasm. It should be taken (inhaled) approximately twenty to thirty minutes before a child participates in any strenuous physical activity to ensure optimal results.

Certain physical activities are more likely to trigger EIB. The sports that require prolonged periods of strenuous activity, such as soccer, tennis, distance cycling, or cross-country running, will more often trigger symptoms compared with activities such as baseball or swimming. With an appropriate plan of action outlined by your child's physician, virtually all children with asthma can be physically active.

The final answer to your question is that your daughter probably has EIB, and no, she most definitely does not need to stop playing soccer.

69. After an asthma attack has subsided, should physical activity be restricted?

The answer to this question is no. Depending on the severity of an asthma attack it may, however, be necessary to temporarily modify you child's physical activities. If the symptoms caused by the activity are mild and last for only a short time, a return to full activity within three to five days is reasonable. On the other hand, if symptoms persist for five to seven days it would be wise to postpone sports such as basketball, soccer, or running for possibly a week or more. The decision regarding the appropriate time to resume unlimited participation in athletic activity should be made jointly by the parents and the child's physician.

It is a myth that children with asthma should avoid physical exertion. In fact, the truth is just the opposite, regular exercise and physical activity should play definite roles in your child's comprehensive asthma management program. Once an asthma attack is under control, it is important to resume normal school, sports, and social activities. Asthma is considered to be under good control when all symptoms have resolved. Breathing should be comfortable. Sleep should be restful and uninterrupted, and cough should have abated, along with wheezing and increased mucus production. Peak flows should have returned to normal or to "personal best" levels.

70. Why is environmental control important in managing my child's asthma?

Between 60% and 80% of children who have asthma are also allergic. If a child's environmental asthma triggers can be identified, and contact with triggers decreased or eliminated, the physician and family will be able to more effectively control the frequency and severity of the child's asthma symptoms. This approach, labeled environmental control, is an important component of a comprehensive asthma management program.

Environmental control is an important component of a comprehensive asthma management program.

For purposes of this discussion, the environment must be divided into its two major components: outdoor and indoor. We all function in both of these physical areas, but unfortunately we can do relatively little as individuals to significantly change the outdoor environment. However, we can as a society make a positive impact in certain areas. One example would be the development of alternative, cleaner energy sources to power our cars, sport utility vehicles, buses, and trucks. This action will help decrease the levels of pollutants in the air and will have a beneficial effect on all people, especially those with respiratory conditions such as asthma, chronic bronchitis, and chronic obstructive pulmonary disease.

Chronic obstructive pulmonary disease

A lung disease of adults which targets the airways. In COPD, the airways and air sacs lose their shape affecting the flow of air.

The allergens that may be present in our homes, day care centers, and schools make up a long list. Sources of potential allergens include dust mites, cockroaches, cats, dogs, gerbils, hamsters, birds, feather pillows and comforters, tobacco smoke, a wood-burning stove or fireplace, carpeting, the heating system, and the presence or absence of air conditioning or air filtering devices.

Dust mites are spider-like insects that are invisible to the naked eye and can only be seen under a microscope. They are so tiny that fifty to seventy dust mites would fit on the head of a pin! They live indoors, and prefer moist environments with greater than 50% relative humidity, along with warmer temperatures near 70°F. Dryer indoor environments with a relative humidity of less than 40% as well as residence at altitude inhibit the growth of dust mites. The highest concentration of these creatures in the home is usually is found in the bedroom. Dust mites' main food supply is human dead skin cells. Bedding, upholstered couches and chairs, and carpets are areas where dust mites thrive. The dust mite allergen is concentrated in the mites' fecal droppings Many children who have asthma are allergic to dust mites. Recommendations for decreasing exposure to dust mites if your child is allergic to them begins with the purchase of special dust mite–proof (impervious) encasings for pillows, mattresses, comforters, and box springs. The single place that your child spends the most time in is his bed, so to further decrease his exposure to dust mite allergen, bed linens and any bedding that is not encased should be washed every week in water that is at least 130°F (55°C). If the water does not reach that temperature, the dust mites are only getting a bath. Dust mites also set up housekeeping in carpeting and in upholstered furniture. If possible, your child's bedroom should have a wood or tile floor and blinds rather than curtains or drapes. Washable cotton throw rugs can be used in the bedroom to minimize dust mite antigen, provided that you do launder the rugs. Stuffed animals or dolls are potential dust mite collectors, and therefore should ideally be kept in a covered toy chest in a room other than the bedroom. Stuffed animals are an abundant source of dust mite allergen, and they are usually right up close to the child's nose and breathing passages! If your child has a favorite stuffed animal, make sure that it is washable and that you wash it in water that is hotter than 130°F at least every two weeks (every week is best) in order to interrupt the mites' reproductive cycle. An alternative to laundering stuffed animals is to place the stuffed animal in a Zip-Lock® bag, seal it, and place the bag in your freezer for 12 hours to 24 hours once a week.

Much to the dismay of allergists, pulmonologists, and pediatricians, most people generally will not relocate a pet who "has become a member of the family." Second-best (and we truly mean "second" best) recommendations include keeping the animal out of your child's bedroom at all times, even when your child is at school or away from home. Dogs can be trained to avoid certain rooms or areas relatively easily, but with cats—animals notorious for their curiosity and lack of obedience—you and your child must make a habit of keeping the child's room strictly secured from the cat's access at all times. Another measure applies if your home has forced air heating. Make sure that the vents in your child's room are covered with appropriate filters. If your cat or dog will cooperate, a weekly bath will help lower the level of animal allergen in your home. These steps may be helpful, but they are truly a distant second best to not having a pet at all.

Smoking should be categorically banned from any household in which a child has asthma of any severity. Increasing numbers of parents are beginning to appreciate this crucial recommendation. Smoke from cigarettes or cigars rarely causes a true allergic reaction; however, the tobacco fumes are major triggers and irritants that definitely will have a negative effect on your child's asthma and adversely affect their lung health. Parents who attempt to limit their smoking to the bathroom, garage, or basement are still smoking indoors where the smoke can be trapped and circulated back into the house. Anywhere air can travel, smoke can travel too—and even limited exposure to second-hand smoke is too much for a child with asthma, particularly if smoke is one of the child's triggers. Parents who smoke in the house are also sending their children the message that their smoking is more important to them than their child's health; this message, unspoken though it may be, can undermine the child's understanding of how important it is to take asthma symptoms seriously and may affect the child's willingness to comply with his or her program of asthma treatment.

Wood-burning fireplaces or stoves are another potential source of trouble for children with asthma. Allergic reactions to burning wood and the release of chemical irritants often cause problems for children with asthma. Mold spores trapped in firewood can also trigger allergic reactions, and various irritating gases can be released as wood burns. A gas-fueled fire is the safest option for any family that feels they must have a fireplace. You must make sure that the fireplace is vented properly, to the outside of your home.

Although down pillows and comforters may be nice to sleep with, some children are allergic to feathers. To be on the safe side, children with asthma should have bedding made of washable cotton or other synthetic filling rather than feathers. Synthetic products are available that are nonallergic and feel similar to down. Primaloft® is one example of a product in this category.

Parents occasionally ask what type of heating system is best for children with asthma. There is no one best answer to this question. A baseboard system may be an allergist's first choice. Forced air heating generally creates an excessively dry environment; however, if an effectively functioning, well-maintained humidifier is built into the system, it should pass muster. A radiator system, especially in large apartment complexes where the ability to regulate the temperature is limited, is probably the least desirable heating system. Radiant and electric systems are expensive, but they are good systems for families with allergies or asthma.

The use of electronic devices to clean or filter the air in your home is something that must be considered when discussing environmental control measures. In a single-family home, a centrally installed system would be best. The appliances that have both a charcoal and a high efficiency particulate air (HEPA) filter are the most effective in removing airborne allergens and irritants. Do not purchase "air purifiers" or ion-

High Efficiency Particulate Air (HEPA) filter

An air filter capable of trapping particles of very small size, including common indoor allergens and even certain microorganisms that pose a risk to human health. HEPA filters are occasionally recommended in the home as part of environmental control measures in treatment of allergy.

izers that emit or produce ozone, a potentially irritating gas, as a byproduct. Ozone, because of its irritant properties, has a real potential to aggravate your child's asthma.

As you can see, there are many areas of environmental control to focus on when discussing the development of a comprehensive asthma management program for your child.

Frank's comment:

Asthma triggers are present almost everywhere you go, that's why environmental control is imperative. However, I draw the line between the overprotective bubble and a comfortable, safe level of normalcy. Growing up, my father was borderline obsessed with "asthma-proofing" my bedroom (which I now appreciate, but it used to drive me insane).

Here are a few minor suggestions of methods and ideas my parents and I used throughout my life. First of all, purchasing a high-quality air purifier for your child's bedroom is potentially helpful in removing airborne allergens. Hypoallergenic under covers for the bed and pillows are beneficial as well. Depending on the severity of the circumstance, you might want to limit the accumulation of "stuff" in your child's room. It's also important to be aware of what's occurring, or the conditions at their school. I attended a brand new middle school from 5th through 8th grade where a great deal of construction was occurring on a daily basis, and from time to time this would aggravate my breathing. Of course this certainly does not mean that you should lock your son/daughter away for the rest of their lives. That could get especially more difficult as they approach their teenage years! The fact is that as long as asthmatic environmental management is instituted for your child, they can live a generally ordinary life.

There are many areas of environmental control to focus on when discussing the development of a comprehensive asthma management program for your child.

Treatment

PART SIX

Recommendations

What is a written asthma action plan?

What is a nebulizer?

What are potential side effects of the asthma medications my daughter is taking?

More . . .

71. What is a written asthma action plan? Should I expect my daughter's doctor to give her one?

Written asthma action plans are important components of a comprehensive approach to the long-term control of your child's asthma. An asthma action plan consists of written management guidelines that provide clear instructions on how to treat your child's asthma when the condition is stable as well as when symptoms are active.

Written asthma self-management and asthma action plans provide clear instructions on how to treat your child's asthma when the condition is stable and when symptoms are active.

The National Asthma Education and Prevention Program (NAEPP) and the Global Initiative for Asthma (GINA) both emphasize patient education and an active partnership among the parents, the patient, and the asthma treatment team in order to provide optimal therapy and ensure the best possible outcome for your child. Asthma self-management is an important component of effective asthma care. Children with asthma should be directly involved in formulating goals of therapy and in developing their asthma action plans as much as is feasible. We believe that a child is who is 9 years old or older should actively and fully participate in their asthma management. The NAEPP advocates that each patient be provided a written individualized daily self-management plan (Table 23) and a written asthma action plan (Figure 5). A written asthma action plan should also be prepared for a child's school and for their camp as well. A sample school asthma action plan is available online at: *www.nhlbi.nih.gov/health/dci/Diseases/Asthma/asthma_actionplan.pdf*

Table 23   A Sample Daily Asthma Self-Management Plan

Asthma Self-Management Plan for: _____

Treatment Goals
- Daytime symptoms: absent (or minimal)
- Nocturnal symptoms: absent (or minimal)
- Lung function: normal (or nearly so)
- Sleep: restful and uninterrupted
- Absences from work or school because of asthma: none
- Participation in sports and team competitions: full
- Regular aerobic exercise: yes
- Exacerbations: addressed and treated promptly and effectively
- Emergency room and hospitalizations: avoided
- Treatment: associated with minimal, if any, side effects
- Additional: _____

_____

_____

Daily Medications

Medicine	Dose	Frequency

Self-Monitoring
Maintain your record in a separate log or diary
- Record symptoms
- Measure peak flow (PEF)
- Record use of maintenance medicine

The NAEPP recommends that the plans be outlined at the patient's first visit, subject to review and revisions at follow-up asthma visits. The daily asthma management plan emphasizes overall goals, medications, patient observations, and self-monitoring during periods of inactive asthma with good control. The action plan provides written guidelines for treating increasing symptomatology and exacerbated asthma.

The key feature of a written asthma action plan is that it is specific for your child. Just as two people with asthma will have different clinical presentations of their disease, they will also require personalized treatment and action plans. The plan for a child whose symptoms usually exacerbate when he has a cold, for example, will likely have instructions about the dose

The asthma action plan is based on your PEF (peak flow) measurements.

Measure and record your PEF.

❑   With any increase in symptoms
❑   When you think your asthma is changing
❑   Each morning after waking up (before any medication)
❑   In the evening, before the evening meal
❑   Before bedtime
❑   Before your inhaler medicine and again 20 minutes later
❑   _____

Record and remember your "personal best" PEF.

Personal best PEF _____

100% of personal best PEF = _____   80% of personal best PEF = _____
50% of personal best PEF =   _____ Less than 50% of personal best PEF = _____

Peak Flow	Symptoms	Treatment	Other
"Green Zone" PEF 80 to 100% GO!	• Comfortable breathing • No symptoms • No nocturnal awakenings	Take: _____ _____	Maintain daily activities.
"Yellow Zone" PEF 60 to 80% CAUTION!	• Uncomfortable • Chest tightness • Cough • Wheeze • Nocturnal symptoms	Add: _____	Increase medicine, treat cold if present, limit exertion. Call MD if not improved.
"Red Zone" PEF < 60% DANGER!	• Very uncomfortable • Limitation on activities • Cough, wheeze	Add: _____ *CONTACT MD or GO TO ER*	Start steroids! Get professional medical opinion.

If the PEF is < 50% and does not rise within 10 minutes of extra medicine as indicated above, if lips and/or fingertips become blue or gray, if you can't walk or talk because of breathlessness and/or wheezing, if breathing is labored, call 911 and proceed immediately to the nearest hospital.

Figure 5   A sample asthma action plan.

of inhaled corticosteroid medication to be taken at the earliest onset of cold symptoms. Another child whose asthma is only rarely triggered by cold symptoms may not need to increase her maintenance controller medication. It is important to remember to review the action plan when you see the doctor in case it becomes necessary to revise some aspect of the recommendations. Sample asthma plans can be found on the Internet; simply use your favorite browser and type "asthma action plan" in the search window.

Despite the strong recommendations of the NAEPP and enthusiastic support from professional medical societies and managed care insurance companies, written asthma plans are not universally popular in the asthma community. When polled, most asthma patients (of all ages!) prefer having a written action plan. The most common reason a person with asthma does not follow a written action plan is simply that the physician never provided one. Studies of written action plans, both here and abroad, have yielded inconsistent results. Some studies report that most patients, especially children, clearly benefit from written asthma plans. The implementation of the action plan should ideally lead to reduced need for hospitalization and to improved asthma control. Other studies suggest that it is not the written plan that improves asthma outcome, but rather the focused attention of the physician and the enhanced interaction between patient and health care provider. In other words, as long as the proper advice on increasing and adjusting medication in asthma is provided, the outcome is improved whether the instructions are given in writing as part of a plan or verbally during an office visit or even over the telephone. If you and your child would like to be provided with an asthma self-management or action plan, you should certainly discuss it with your child's doctor at your next visit.

Recommendations

72. What is the correct way to use a metered-dose inhaler (MDI)?

Metered-dose inhalers (MDIs) are convenient, highly portable, and very reliable devices designed to deliver medicine in an aerosolized form through inhalation. MDIs are conceptually similar to dry powder inhalers (DPIs) (discussed in Question 57). Although MDIs and DPIs both allow the delivery of accurate, pre-measured doses of medicine directly to the respiratory passages, they also have some basic, fundamental differences. MDIs use a propellant to push the medicine out of its dosing canister. All MDIs on the market in the United States are manually activated rather than breath activated, except for the Maxair® Autohaler®, which is the only breath activated MDI. Manual activation means that the medicine is released from the device when the user presses down on the canister. Breath activated means that the medicine is automatically released as the user inhales deeply. Because most MDIs are manually activated, their proper use is technically more challenging and requires more coaching than is the case for DPIs.

The correct way to use the MDI is best demonstrated by your child's physician. There are two techniques for best use: the open-mouth and the closed-mouth techniques. All MDIs come with directions. The directions, or what your pharmacist calls the manufacturer's package insert, describe the closed-mouth technique. Asthma specialists generally prefer to teach the open-mouth method of using the MDI because they believe it improves the delivery of medicine and favors the inhalation of the more desirable, smaller released particles. A description of the open-mouth MDI technique follows; keep reading!

The correct way to use an MDI is best demonstrated by your child's physician.

MDIs should be kept at room temperature and should not be subjected to sustained temperatures less than 59°F or more than 77°F. MDIs should be stored in a vertical or upright position with the mouthpiece down when not in use. If you notice that the plastic mouthpiece becomes coated with a whitish powder, pull the metal MDI canister out of the plastic mouthpiece and rinse the mouthpiece under warm tap water until it looks clean. Make sure the mouthpiece is completely dry before reinserting the metal canister. The plastic part can be air-dried. Each MDI comes with specific "cleaning" instructions and they are listed in the package insert which should be dispensed by your pharmacy.

All MDIs should ideally be allowed to reach room temperature before use. If you carry your child's fast-acting quick-relief MDI with you and you are outdoors on an especially cold day, place it in an inner pocket close to your body rather than in a handbag or backpack. Never leave an MDI in the glove compartment or trunk of your car on a hot summer day; its contents are under pressure and can explode in very hot environments (120°F or more).

The general concept of the MDI is to trigger the release of medicine from the MDI while simultaneously inhaling the medication into "empty" lungs. The basic technique consists of (1) an initial exhalation to empty the lungs, (2) release of a puff of medication (the "actuation") to coincide with a full, steady, deep inhalation that lasts 3 to 5 seconds, followed by (3) breath holding (the "hold") to allow the medicine to deposit deep in the lung. Of course, it is extremely difficult to time the puff of medication exactly to the start of the inhalation, so our standard advice is to start inhaling and as you start to inhale, release the puff ("actuate"), continuing to slowly inhale for 3 to 5 seconds, then hold that breath to a count of 10 and slowly exhale. The most common technical error we observe as patients learn to use MDIs is when they stop the inhalation at the time that they actuate the MDI!

The technically most difficult part of learning to use an MDI for children as well as adults thus involves the coordination of inhalation and release of the medicine from the canister. Because of this, your child's physician will likely prescribe the MDIs with a spacer device that attaches directly to the MDI mouthpiece. A spacer facilitates inhalation of the medicine from the MDI. As a rule of thumb, children younger than 5 years of age should use an MDI with a spacer device that is fitted with a facemask, and children older than 5 years should be prescribed a dedicated spacer device with a mouthpiece for use with their MDI (see Table 24). Spacer devices are discussed in detail in Question 73.

MD Turbo® is a novel medical device designed to facilitate use of MDIs. It is available by perscription from your child's doctor and works with many different manufacturers' MDIs. You first load your MDI inhaler into the MD Turbo® and then as your child inhales through the mouthpiece, a puff of medication is released on demand, automatically. The device thus "converts" your patient activated MDI into a breath activated MDI. Since you no longer have to press down on the canister of the MDI to actuate it, the MD Turbo® overcomes the frequent problems of coordinating the press and breath-in maneuver. The device also incorporates a dose counter that tells you how many puffs you have taken from your MDI.

You will, of course, need to supervise and assist your child as he or she learns to master MDIs. The information that follows explains the correct way to use an MDI. Even though your child younger than 12 years of age will likely use an MDI with an attached facemask or spacer, we find it useful for you to understand proper open-mouth technique. Before using the MDI, remove the cap from the mouthpiece. Your child ideally should be standing to use the inhaler. If your child prefers to be seated, make sure that he or she sits upright. The inhaler should be held straight up with the mouthpiece at the bottom. Many people find it most comfortable to hold the MDI with their thumb at the lowermost portion and their middle finger on the topmost metal portion of the MDI canister. Next, shake the MDI canister to mix the medicine. After shaking the MDI, position the mouthpiece two to three finger widths (one to two inches) in front of your child's open mouth. Your child should tilt his or her head back very slightly and gently breathe out. Once he or she has emptied the lungs, press on the MDI and, as simultaneously as possible, your child should take a slow, deep breath and keep breathing inward for at least five seconds. Once your child has inhaled fully, the breath should be held to allow the medicine to penetrate throughout the bronchial passageways. Your child should try to hold his or her breath for ten seconds, and then exhale and resume normal breathing. If the doctor prescribed a second puff of medication, your child may be instructed to wait a minute or more between doses. The MDI-delivered medicine should go into the lungs; consequently, it not should irritate your child's throat or cause him or her to cough, nor should it land on the tongue and cause a "strange" taste. It is important that your child learn to use the prescribed MDI correctly (Table 24). Make sure you ask your child's physician any questions you may have about the way your child is using the MDI. We find it very useful to watch our patients' MDI technique during an office visit. A well-placed suggestion can make a big difference. Remember that mastering good MDI technique involves a learning curve and, with proper instruction and supervision, even young children can use MDI-delivered asthma medication.

Table 24   Metered-Dose Inhaler: Common Errors in Technique

Forgetting to shake the MDI canister before use

Sitting hunched over when inhaling your medicine

Blocking the MDI mouthpiece with your tongue or your teeth.

Releasing the puff of medicine either before ("too soon") or after ("too late") you have started to inhale deeply ("poor coordination" pattern)

Taking in too shallow a breath

Forgetting to hold your breath for at least 10 seconds after inhaling the medicine

Neglecting to rinse your mouth after using the inhaled corticosteroid MDI

Immersing the canister in water

Forgetting to replace the MDI canister before the expiration date marked on the label, even if it is not empty

Continuing to use the MDI even though all the doses have been dispensed from it

73. What is a spacer device, and why should I buy one for my child?

A spacer is a device prescribed with a metered-dose inhaler (MDI). Holding chambers (HCs) are an especially useful type of spacer device. The benefits of using a holding chamber are at least threefold. They eliminate one of the major challenges in using an MDI properly: coordinating the almost-simultaneous discharge of the medicine and the need to inhale. They make it easier to use MDIs, and for children under the age of 5, they are generally essential; children that young aren't usually capable of timing the inhalation correctly without it. Holding chamber use improves the delivery of the medication into the bronchial passageways. Holding chambers reduce potential side effects such as cough, hoarseness, thrush, and throat irritation related to inhaled steroid medicine settling in the throat. A higher concentration of the medicine goes where it is needed and less goes where it is not. You first press on the MDI canister to release the medicine into the device, and a second or so later, your child inhales that same puff of medication from the holding chamber.

A spacer is a device prescribed with a metered-dose inhaler (MDI) that improves the delivery of the medication into the bronchial passageways.

Spacers, in general, and holding chambers in particular, make it easier for you or your child with asthma to use an MDI effectively. They are recommended for children or anyone who experiences difficulty coordinating deep inhalation and activation of the MDI, and are also indicated when MDI corticosteroids are prescribed. In fact, one inhaled corticosteroid, Azmacort® (the brand of triamcinolone distributed by Kos Pharmaceuticals), is sold with an incorporated spacer device so that anyone using it must inhale the medication through its spacer.

Within the next year, metered-dose inhalers used for the treatment of asthma will use HFA as the propellent rather than CFC, which has been banned (see Question 55). The significance of this fact is that the HFA MDIs must use a non-electrostatic holding chamber. Currently, there is one non-electrostatic holding chamber (HC) commercially available in North America, the Vortex® manufactured by Pari Respiratory Equipment Company. This device is made of aluminum. The aluminum surface does not attract the aerosolized particles, therefore more medication is available to be inhaled into the lungs.

Kerrin's comment:

Now that my son is getting a bit older, his allergy specialist prescribed an albuterol MDI with a spacer for him to use when he needs it. The inhaler fits right into one end of the tube, and there is a soft rubber-rimmed mask that fits over the nose and mouth on the other end. And rather than sitting for fifteen to twenty minutes with the nebulizer, this delivers the medicine in twelve breaths (six breaths for each of two pushes on the MDI canister). It's much more convenient to use because I don't have to look for an electrical socket and a place to sit comfortably for fifteen to twenty minutes with a squirmy child.

74. What is the correct way to use a dry powder inhaler (DPI)?

Dry powder inhalers (DPIs) deliver asthma medicine as fine particles of powder. As discussed in Question 57, many types of DPIs are available. Every DPI delivery device has unique instructions for optimal use. When your child's physician prescribes a DPI as asthma treatment, the physician should both demonstrate the correct way for your child to use the device and provide appropriate instructions for its use. When you fill the prescription, make sure that the dispensing pharmacist includes the directions provided by the manufacturer. Medication delivered via a DPI device can be considered for children with asthma who are 4 to 5 years of age and older.

Although each DPI is unique and comes with its own set of specific instructions, all DPIs share some similarities. They are prized for their ease of use, reliability, efficiency, and convenience.

All DPIs are breath-activated and contain medication in a dry powder form. It is very important that the medication remain dry. You should not, for example, store an opened DPI in a moist environment, such as in a humid bathroom. Your child should also never exhale into the mouthpiece of a DPI, because the moisture in the exhaled breath can affect the effectiveness of the medication contained in the device. A DPI is designed to automatically release an exact pre-measured dose of medicine as your child inhales. The technique your child uses while breathing in (inhaling) helps determine how effectively the medicine penetrates into the bronchial passageways. The actual technique basically consists of inhaling the medicine through the DPI mouthpiece starting with empty lungs, and then holding the breath before exhaling and breathing normally. Your child begins by: (1) breathing out (exhaling) to empty his or her lungs, then (2) breathing in (inhaling) fairly rapidly from the mouthpiece, followed by (3) holding his or her breath for approximately ten seconds. The concept is: "out-in-hold!"

To use a DPI correctly, the parent or the child must first "load" the DPI with a pre-measured dose of medicine, either by rotating and clicking the device, advancing a small lever, or physically inserting a powder-containing capsule into a specially designed groove in the device depending on which type of DPI has been prescribed. Once the medicine is "loaded" or primed, your child should then take a breath of room air and fully, but gently, exhale it into the room. When the lungs feel "empty" and all the air has been "blown out," your child should place his lips around the DPI's mouthpiece and take a full, steady, deep breath, inhaling the medicine until he cannot breathe in any further. The final step requires that your child hold his breath with his "lungs full of medicine." Children should breath-hold for at least ten seconds before exhaling (count to ten in your head or even out loud!). After the count of ten, your child should remove the DPI mouthpiece from his lips and let his breath out. Children should always remember to exhale into the room and not into the DPI device.

The reason children need to hold their breath after taking the inhaled dose of medicine is to allow the medicine to penetrate into the air passages. As they hold their breath, there is no movement of air in the lungs—which is important because it allows the asthma medicine to settle in the lungs long enough to work effectively. Exhaling too soon means your child will not get the full benefit of the medicine.

You should become familiar with the specific DPI device prescribed for your child. Read the manufacturer's "Instructions for Patient Use" insert provided with the product. Ask the treating physician any questions you may have. Encourage your child, who is the patient after all, to read the materials that you have already reviewed. Even a young child can look at the illustrations provided alongside the written instructions to get an idea of how to correctly use the dry powder device. We often ask our patients to bring their DPI with them to their appointment so they can demonstrate their technique. We are then able to assess the effectiveness of this technique and make specific suggestions, if appropriate.

Note that each DPI not only looks unique but also has specific characteristics. For example, the disposable Diskus® device is packaged in a foil pouch, and the manufacturer states that it should be used or discarded within one month of opening to prevent the medicine from drying out. The Diskus® also has a unique dosage counter that shows how many doses of medicine remain in the device. The numbers in the Diskus® dose indicator turn red when only five doses are left to alert you to refill your prescription. When the "0" is displayed, your Diskus® is empty. Children should always keep the inhaler in a horizontal position during use. If they are left handed, they may find it more comfortable and natural to turn the Diskus® device over and use with the label parallel to the floor, facing "upside down", so that the lever is easier to click into position with the left thumb while holding the device in their left hand. The Diskus® should be closed to cover the mouthpiece after each use and does not require any other maintenance or

Parents should become familiar with the specific DPI device prescribed for their child.

cleaning. Never exhale into a Diskus® to avoid introducing moisture into the device and inactivating the medication.

The Turbuhaler® is a DPI delivery device similar to the Diskus® in that it too comes preloaded with medicine. However, rather than needing to push a lever away from you to prepare the dose, the Turbuhaler® requires that you rotate the base of the device all the way to the right and back to the left until it clicks. The Turbuhaler® does not actually display the amount of doses remaining in the device, but it alerts you when twenty doses remain. A red mark appears at the top of the window when you are down to twenty doses. When the marking is at the bottom of the window, the Turbuhaler® is empty. The Turbuhaler® must always be re-capped after use to keep it clean and dry; the mouthpiece can be wiped with a dry cloth, but the device should not be washed.

The Twisthaler® is another device that also provides a month of preloaded medication. The user twists while removing the device's cap, preparing the next dose for inhalation. The Twisthaler® not only counts down as the medicine is used up but also firmly locks the cap into place after the last dose is used, preventing the user from using an empty device.

The Diskhaler®, Aerolizer®, and Handihaler® devices require that you load the DPI before use. The Diskhaler® holds up to eight doses of medicine at a time and requires simple but regular maintenance and cleaning. The Aerolizer® and Handihaler® accept only one dose at a time. The Rotahaler® similarly requires insertion of a dose before use and regular cleaning. Although it is one of the first DPIs developed for patient use, the Rotahaler® has been replaced in practice by newer DPIs.

75. How can I tell when my child's asthma inhaler is nearly empty?

It is easy to know if a dry powder inhaler (DPI) is empty or not because DPIs are specifically designed with counters that keep track of how many doses remain in the inhaler and remind you when to refill your child's prescription. Preloaded DPIs, such as the Diskus®, are dispensed by your pharmacist in a moisture-protective foil wrapper. Most preloaded DPI must be discarded within thirty days of opening the foil wrapper regardless of whether or not the counter registers "0" doses. Some medicines in DPI form, such as mometasone in the Twisthaler® delivery system, have a slightly longer shelf life of forty-five days after opening. The "Instructions for Patients" that come with the prescribed DPI will specify how long a DPI can be kept before it has to be replaced with fresh medicine.

Metered-dose inhalers (MDIs), with one exception, do not have built-in dose counters. The exception, a new formulation of albuterol called Ventolin® HFA, has a novel counter incorporated into the mouthpiece and first became available in the summer of 2006. Various strategies have been advocated over the years to help indicate when an MDI is empty or nearly empty. One suggestion that we mention because we advise against it involves removing the metal MDI canister from its plastic mouthpiece and dropping it into a tall glass of water. If the metal canister sank to the bottom, it was supposedly close to full. If it settled halfway to the surface, you still had plenty of medicine. If it started to bob close to the surface, it was time to get a refill. MDI manufacturers and the FDA are strongly opposed to immersing the metal MDI canister in water, and therefore most doctors advise against floating the canister under any circumstances. Also note that you cannot tell if an MDI is empty by shaking it; it may still contain propellant even after the active medicine is used up.

Technically speaking, the only way to be certain that an MDI still contains medicine is to actually count each dose used. Small external counters that fit in the palm of your hand, like the counters used to count attendance at museums or concerts, can be clicked each time the MDI is used, an accurate but not too practical plan! The truth is that, except in the case of the Ventolin® HFA inhaler with an incorporated dose counter, there is no method of MDI dose counting that is both reliable and convenient. Instead of trying to guess when your child's MDI is completely empty, we suggest that you estimate ahead of time when you will need to replace the MDI. Your estimate should take into account (1) how many doses or actuations the MDI contains and (2) how frequently your child uses the MDI medication. If a youngster is prescribed an MDI that contains 200 puffs of medicine for example, and he takes two puffs of the medication three times a day, then he will be using a total of six [2 puffs x 3 times = 6] puffs daily. Given that the new MDI comes with 200 puffs, it should provide enough medicine for about 30 days [take 200 and divide it by 6]. You can also ask your pulmonary doctor or pharmacist to help you estimate when you will need to obtain an MDI refill. Basically, you divide the total number of doses in the full MDI by the total number of daily doses you anticipate your child will use to determine how long the MDI will last. Consider recording the date in your calendar or personal digital assistant (PDA) so you remember to contact your pharmacist a day or two in advance of the date the MDI is anticipated to be empty. Finally, note that the newest MDIs that use hydrofluoroalkane (HFA) propellants may have special requirements. The CFC-free Ventolin® HFA, which is often prescribed as a fast-acting quick-relief asthma medication, should be discarded and replaced after two hundred puffs are released from the MDI or if 2 months have passed since the sealed, moisture-protective foil wrapper was opened, whichever comes first.

Actuation

The action that releases a dose of medication from a metered-dose inhaler(MDI).

75. What is a nebulizer?

A nebulizer is a device powered by either electrical current or batteries that creates a fine mist of medicine particles that are easily inhaled into the lungs' breathing passages. It is uncomplicated in its method of operation. A short piece of specialized plastic tubing attaches the motor-driven compressor (power source) on one end to the to the nebulizer proper at the other. The compressor sends air through the tubing that connects to the nebulizer's receptacle (or "cup") where the medication in liquid form is placed. When the machine is turned on, the air travels though the tubing and is forced through the liquid medicine in the nebulizer cup to create a finely dispersed medicated mist. Breathing the mist through an attached facemask or a mouthpiece permits delivery of medicine to the bronchial passageways. Some people use the term "breathing machine" interchangeably with the term "nebulizer." Strictly speaking, the nebulizer is the device at the other end of the tubing from the compressor, and not the entire set-up. That said, most people, including doctors, refer to the entire machine—the compressor, tubing, medication cup, and mouthpiece (or facemask)—collectively as "the nebulizer."

Many parents wrongly become upset if a physician suggests that they should have a nebulizer at home because they think it is a sign that the child's condition is more severe than it may actually be. If your child's physician has advised a nebulizer, remember that it is merely an alternative method of delivering needed medication. Many children with asthma require steroids or bronchodilators, which must be delivered by inhalation. The use of a metered-dose inhaler (MDI) with or without a spacer device or facemask is the more commonly prescribed method of delivering therapeutic aerosols. However, we must stress that the recommendation that you have a nebulizer at home does not necessarily mean that your child's asthma has become more severe. Your child is not "being hooked up to a machine" because his or her condition has

A nebulizer is a device powered by either electrical current or batteries that creates a fine mist of medicine particles that are easily inhaled into the lungs' breathing passages.

Recommendations

worsened. Yes, a nebulizer is an electrical device, but keep in mind that it is a valid and often very useful alternative to using medication delivered by an MDI or DPI ("puffer") device. A nebulizer transforms the asthma medicine in liquid form into an aerosol that penetrates deeply into your child's lungs with every inspiration. The widespread use of portable nebulizers has made it possible for parents to treat asthma exacerbations at home, often eliminating the need for emergency room visits and possible hospitalization.

A special caution concerns nebulizer use in toddlers and young children. A child younger than 5 years must use a facemask when nebulized medication is administered. To obtain maximal benefit from the treatment, the facemask must create a tight seal over your child's nose and mouth. Delivering nebulized medicine using what has been called the blow-by technique is totally ineffective. The blow-by method attempts to deliver medication by holding the bulb that contains the medicine under the child's nose and mouth, with the hope that it will reach the lungs. Unfortunately, it does not work! The blow-by technique does not require that you hold a mask to the child's face, so although a parent may believe they are still treating their child's asthma effectively, the fact is that only insignificant amounts of medicine reach the breathing passages.

The medications used in the treatment of asthma, available either in liquid form for nebulization or through an MDI device, include bronchodilators (albuterol, Xopenex®, pirbu terol),corticosteroids (Pulmicort® Respules®), and mast-cell stabilizers (Intal®).

Kerrin's comment:

My son was first given his nebulizer when he was about 8 months old. He quickly got used to it and will now ask for a treatment if he's feeling uncomfortable. We have learned that it is a good idea to bring the nebulizer with us (and plenty of albuterol) if we may be going to a place where a trigger might be present, such as a friend's house or an outdoor event. We also know it is important to remember to pack it when going on vacation, along with enough medication to last if my son gets a respiratory illness that could potentially trigger symptoms.

77. How do I use a nebulizer?

Many medications indicated in asthma treatment are produced in a form suitable for nebulization. The two major types of nebulizers are jet nebulizers and ultrasonic nebulizers. Most pulmonologists prefer jet nebulizers for their patients as they produce medication particles to more uniform size. If Pulmicort® Respules®, an inhaled steroid preparation, has been prescribed for your child, it must be administered through a jet nebulizer only. The Respules® should not be delivered through an ultrasonic nebulizer.

Several studies have shown that each brand or variety of nebulizer available in the marketplace has different medication-delivery profiles. Although all nebulizers work similarly, you should fully familiarize yourself with the specific nebulizer that your child's physician prescribes. Read all directions for its use and maintenance carefully. Many nebulizer manufacturers maintain Internet sites for their products, and the Web can be a good source of information for patients.

To use a nebulizer, you will need to attach the plastic tubing to the nebulizer, your child must inhale the nebulized medication (treatment), which should take between ten and twenty minutes, and then you should clean and prepare the nebulizer for the next use, cleaning it more thoroughly every other day according to the manufacturer's directions.

Here are some general guidelines on how to use your nebulizer. Babies and young children will need to use a special mask rather than a mouthpiece. Understand that your particular machine has specific instructions for its proper use.

Recommendations

First, always collect all equipment and medicine you will require, including the nebulizer, tubing, medicine, and compressor. Wash your hands. Use a clean nebulizer and fill the medication cup with one dose of your child's medicine as directed by the physician. Connect the air tubing between the nebulizer and the compressor, along with a finger valve if your setup requires one. Attach a mouthpiece (or mask) to the nebulizer. Turn the compressor on and check that the nebulizer is producing a medication mist. Your child should then place his or her lips around the mouthpiece and stabilize the mouthpiece between the teeth, or you should gently apply the mask to your child's face, ensuring a good seal. Remember to hold the nebulizer upright to avoid spills and to increase its effectiveness. Your child should ideally breathe gently and calmly. Try to teach your child to inhale deeply for three to five seconds before holding his or her breath for up to ten seconds (and you should count) and then exhaling normally. If the nebulizer has a finger valve, you should cover the hole in the finger valve while your child inhales, and uncover the valve when he or she exhales. Repeat the process of drawing deep breaths, followed by breath holds, until the nebulizer begins to make sputtering sounds. The sputtering sound signals that your child's treatment is finished.

When all medication solution has been nebulized, disassemble the nebulizer setup. Wash all the parts, except for the tubing and finger valve, in liquid dish soap and water. Rinse in tap water and shake off any excess water droplets. Reconnect the different parts and run the compressor to dry the nebulizer. Wait until the nebulizer is completely dry before storing it. If your child uses a nebulizer daily, you should also perform a more in-depth cleaning every forty-eight hours or so. When doing so, you should wash your hands first. Then, put aside the tubing and valve, and prepare a fresh solution of distilled white vinegar and hot water by using one part white vinegar to three parts hot water (one-quarter white vinegar to three-quarters hot water). Soak all parts of the nebulizer (except the tubing and mask) in the vinegar and hot water solution for sixty minutes. After an hour, remove the nebulizer parts and rinse them under running water. Throw away the soaking solution. After rinsing in fresh water, shake off any excess water droplets. Reconnect the different parts of the setup and run the compressor to dry the nebulizer. Wait until the nebulizer is completely dry before storing it. Make sure to find out if the compressor unit you are using requires specific maintenance or cleaning.

78. Is medication in nebulized form more effective than in an inhaler?

The answer is: no, not necessarily, and not usually. Several studies have shown that inhaled asthma medication in metered-dose inhaler (MDI) form is just as effective as that administered through a nebulizer, provided a spacer device such as a holding chamber is used with the MDI and the patient has mastered appropriate technique. MDIs are inexpensive, basically maintenance free, highly portable, and very convenient. Nebulizers are more cumbersome, need a power source, and require frequent cleaning. The same medicine that can be administered in two or three minutes using an MDI will take close to fifteen minutes with nebulization.

There are a few specific situations when a nebulizer rather than an MDI–spacer setup might be considered. Babies and very young children who are too young to learn MDI technique should receive their medicine through nebulization using a facemask. Some children can be taught correct MDI technique when they are of kindergarten age, particularly if there is a motivated adult in the home to supervise and encourage the child. Young children with persistent poorly controlled asthma should, under the guidance of a physician, have a nebulizer at home for emergency use. Any child who is unable to use an MDI, perhaps because of a physical or neurologic impairment, can receive asthma medicine through a nebulizer. Finally, some children who have very poor lung function may be unable to inhale deeply enough to benefit

Several studies have shown that inhaled asthma medication in metered-dose inhaler (MDI) form is just as effective as that administered through a nebulizer.

Recommendations

from using an MDI and therefore should switch to a nebulizer. The last scenario is unusual in a young person who only has asthma; however, a child who has both cystic fibrosis and asthma could fall into this category.

79. Should my daughter use a metered-dose inhaler (MDI) as a preventative measure before playing sports?

The answer depends on the severity of your daughter's asthma. If she has controlled or mild intermittent asthma, for example, and if exercise triggers symptoms of asthma, such as cough, mucus production, and uncomfortable breathing, then using an MDI before strenuous physical activity may well be indicated. Treatment options in this situation include a short-acting β_2 agonist, such as albuterol, and inhaled cromolyn (Intal®).

For many school-aged children, exercise is arguably the single most common asthma trigger. These children with inadequately controlled asthma often experience variable cough, wheezing, and breathlessness with exertion and exercise. Exercise-induced asthma (EIA) is a clinically different phenomenon. EIA does not reflect inadequately controlled asthma. Some physicians consider it a subtype of asthma, whereas others view it as a possible precursor to asthma and prefer the descriptive term exercise-induced bronchospasm (EIB) when reporting exercise-related symptoms in a child with underlying asthma in order to clearly emphasize that EIA is a separate clinical entity (see Questions 66 and 67).

Individuals with exercise-induced bronchospasm (EIB) experience respiratory symptoms during and after aerobic exercise. The symptoms may include cough, wheezing, and shortness of breath, along with chest discomfort. The symptoms usually develop within five to ten minutes after exercise begins and often lessen or even resolve altogether as exercise is continued and repeated. In some individuals, the symptoms of EIB may begin shortly after the physical activity ends. Treatment includes proper attention to warm-up and cool-down maneuvers, and prescription medication. Another "trick" aims to decrease the inhalation of cold air: encourage your daughter to breathe through her nose rather than though her mouth so as to warm and humidify the ambient air before it reaches the bronchial passages. You could also consider asking her to wear a facemask or cover her mouth and nose with a scarf (tucking the ends carefully inside her jacket) if she likes to participate in outdoor winter sports, such as skiing or skating. Medicines effective in treating EIB include oral leukotriene modifiers; inhaled, short-acting β_2 agonists; and inhaled cromolyn. If inhalers are prescribed, they should be taken approximately twenty to thirty minutes before the warm-up routine.

80. What are the potential side effects of the asthma medicines my daughter is taking?

The potential side effects of your daughter's asthma medicines depend on the specific medicines she is taking. Remember that each child's asthma treatment regimen is individualized. The medicines your daughter uses currently may be different from those that she will require next year. Asthma is an episodic and variable condition with alternating periods of increased symptoms and quiescent symptoms. Visualize asthma as a kind of wave, with ebbs and flows. A 6-year-old who wheezes when she gets sick with a respiratory virus or cold will require different asthma medicines as compared to a 13-year-old who has cough, mucus, and wheeze most days of the week. Because all people with asthma are different one from another, treatments also vary.

Asthma medications, when used as directed, generally have minimal side effects. One of the major asthma treatment goals of the National Asthma Education and Prevention Program (NAEPP) and the Global Initiative for Asthma (GINA) is to prescribe treatments that have either no or minimal side effects. Any medication has a potential to cause a "side effect" in a certain percentage of people. Side effects can be defined as unanticipated symptoms that are caused by the treatment, but are unrelated to the primary treatment effect of the medicine.

Each child's asthma treatment regimen is individualized.

For example, the antibiotic prescribed to cure an infection may also cause stomach upset and diarrhea. The main reason for prescribing the antibiotic was its ability to cure the infection; the stomach pains and diarrhea are the unanticipated side effects. This definition does not include the effects of an overdose and also distinguishes a drug intolerance from a side effect. Every medicine has a unique chemical formula, and chemically similar medicines tend to exhibit similar side effect and safety profiles. Side effects are a function of the dose of medicine, the way the medicine is administered, and unique patient characteristics. Physicians will prescribe the lowest dose of a medicine that achieves the desired clinical benefit, partly to decrease the possible occurrence of side effects. Because the preferred method of administering asthma medications is by inhalation (see Question 53) directly into the breathing passages, they tend to cause fewer generalized side affects than medicines taken orally.

To get back to your question regarding your daughter's medicines, bronchodilator medication, such as the β_2 agonists (inhalers, pills, and liquids), has as its most frequent side effect stimulation of the heartbeat. β_2 agonist bronchodilator medicines in oral form (as opposed to inhalers in particular) often cause generalized stimulation, especially in younger children. Parents report that some younger children get highly active and agitated ("hyper") when they need to take oral β_2 agonists.

The most common adverse effect of inhaled corticosteroids involves the throat, so if your daughter is prescribed inhaled corticosteroids, she should always rinse her mouth after every dose of inhaled corticosteroids. Rinsing helps prevent throat irritation and the development of thrush. Using a spacer device if a metered-dose inhaler (MDI) is prescribed also significantly reduces throat irritation and hoarseness, as reviewed in Question 73. Oral (pill or liquid) corticosteroids have significant side effects if used in high doses or for longer periods, and are more fully discussed in Question 58. Oral leukotrienes have minimal side effects, which is in part why they are FDA approved for use in children as young as 2 years of age. Most dispensing pharmacies usually include a printout with your child's prescription explaining how the medicine works and what side effects can occur. If you suspect that your child is experiencing a side effect from any of her asthma medicines, you must contact the doctor. The physician is knowledgeable about the medication and will, if necessary, adjust the dosage or perhaps even change your daughter's medicine altogether. You should never stop your child's asthma medicine without first having a discussion with your child's physician.

81. What are the newest asthma medicines?

Scientific advances in the basic understanding of asthma at the molecular and genetic levels continue to energize research and the development of new and more effective asthma treatments. Bringing a novel asthma medication to market is an arduous, complicated, and expensive process. It can take many years and hundreds of millions of dollars before your doctor can write a prescription for the newest drug. Effectiveness and safety are the primary concerns of the pharmaceutical industry and the federal agencies responsible for licensing any drug. All medicines must go through a rigorous approval program before they become available for use by the general public.

Asthma is a condition of great interest to physicians, researchers, epidemiologists, and public health experts. The modern approach to asthma treatment includes an accurate classification schema, patient and caregiver education, the institution of stepwise therapy with emphasis on trigger identification and avoidance, and the all-important role of anti-inflammatory medicines. Dry powder inhalers (DPIs) are a recent development, as is the design of novel medication based on the basic science of asthma. The leukotriene antagonist medications, for example, were designed based on the specific study of leukotrienes, which are produced in greater numbers in allergic and asthmatic persons. A better understanding of asthma and allergy at the molecular level has recently resulted in a new class of medicine referred to as IgE blockers (Table 25).

Recommendations

Table 25   The First in a New Class of Asthma Treatments: IgE Blockers

Xolair® (Omalizumab), a medication that binds immunoglobulin E, is the prototype of a new and unique class of asthma treatment, the IgE blockers

---

Omazilumab is:
- a humanized monoclonal antibody
- administered by injection, right under the skin (subcutaneous)
- taken every 2 to 4 weeks under direct medical supervision
- dosed based on the patient's IgE level and weight
- FDA approved for use in patients age 12 years and older
  (as of this writing)
- indicated in adolescents and adults with
    severe persistent asthma who have significant allergy (and asthma)
    a positive skin test to a specific allergen
    a positive RAST test to a specific allergen
    asthma poorly controlled despite inhaled corticosteroids
- *not* used in acute or emergency treatment of an exacerbation

---

Asthma is a condition of great interest to physicians, researchers, epidemiologists, and public health experts.

Anaphylaxis

The most severe form of an allergic reaction or response. If untreated, anaphylaxis can be fatal.

Immunoglobulin E (IgE), first identified in the mid-1960s, is a protein produced by the body. IgE is an antibody and is normally produced in minute quantities. It circulates in the bloodstream in very small amounts. Under certain conditions, however, the body's (and blood or serum) level of IgE can rise significantly. High serum IgE levels have, for example, been associated with persistent wheezing, eczema, allergy, and bronchial hyperresponsiveness. IgE plays a pivotal role in allergy, asthma, and other atopic diseases, such as eczema, seasonal allergic rhinitis, food allergy, anaphylaxis, and hives. To better understand the central role of IgE, it is important to review our current knowledge of the physiologic mechanisms involved in allergic reactions.

When a person becomes "allergic" to a specific substance or protein, it is the result of a phenomenon called "sensitization." In order to become sensitized, prior exposure is necessary. A child may become sensitized after the first exposure, or not until the tenth exposure. This characteristic varies from one individual to the next. There is no way to determine if or when any one child will become sensitized. Although many people are "allergic" to something, fortunately not everyone has the ability or potential to react allergically.

Consider, for example, two siblings who live in a home with a cat. One child has no allergic symptoms, whereas the other child experiences itchy eyes, runny nose, chest tightness, and wheezing whenever she is in the house, particularly if she is in direct contact with the cat. The second child has become sensitized to the cat, and she has developed symptoms of allergic rhinitis and allergic asthma triggered by her allergy to the cat. Her body has produced anti-cat IgE antibodies, and these IgE antibodies are what cause the symptoms of sneeze, cough, and wheezing. It is straightforward to measure any child's total serum IgE level with a simple blood test. An elevated serum IgE level directed against a specific antigen indicates that sensitization against that antigen has occurred, but it does not automatically indicate that an allergy to that antigen is present as well. In fact, it is possible for a child to have both an elevated total serum IgE level in the blood and no allergy symptoms at all. For this reason, measurement of the IgE level alone may not be helpful in assessing the child's potential to have allergy symptoms. If a child has a history suggesting an allergic reaction to peanut butter on the other hand, and her specific anti-peanut IgE antibody is high, then it is a safe bet that she is allergic to peanuts. Remember (see Question 34) that before you can state that someone is "allergic" to something, both a positive test for the suspected allergen and a history of a response are required. Either alone is sufficient to confirm allergy.

Allergy specialists have two types of tests at their disposal to determine the presence of specific for IgE antibodies: an indirect method via blood testing (RAST® or ImmunoCAP®) and direct skin tests (prick-puncture or intradermal test). In our earlier example of the child who is allergic to her cat, we would expect that diagnostic testing would show her to have an elevated total IgE blood measurement, a high level of cat-directed IgE (anti-cat IgE) in the blood on RAST® or ImmunoCAP® testing, and a positive skin test to cat allergen.

Scientists have been able to precisely analyze various effects of IgE at the cellular level in humans. Researchers have been able to map out how the IgE, in concert with specialized white blood cells (such as macrophages, T cells, B cells, and activated mast cells) collectively termed effector cells, interact and release substances or "mediators" that create the typical symptoms of an allergic response. The sophisticated research has not only advanced our understanding of how allergy and asthma develop, but has also suggested pathways for new asthma and allergy medications. In particular, a novel medication, omalizumab (Xolair®), was developed specifically for use in patients with IgE-mediated asthma. The U.S. Food and Drug Administration (FDA) approved omalizumab in June of 2003. Omalizumab treats asthma via a unique and novel mechanism as compared to that of existing asthma medicines. Omalizumab actually binds the IgE circulating in the body. The IgE is bound by the medication and thus cannot interact with effector cells. Since bound IgE is not available for interaction with effector cells, release of the mediators responsible for the development of asthma symptoms is inhibited. Omalizumab became available by prescription in the United States in July of 2003. It is approved by the FDA for treating moderate persistent or severe persistent allergic asthma in young people aged 12 years and older, adolescents, and adults who meet two specific criteria. One is the presence of a positive skin test or RAST® blood test for a year-round allergen, such as dust mite or mold. The second criterion requires that inhaled corticosteroid treatment be ineffective in adequately controlling the patient's asthmatic symptomatology. Omalizumab therapy requires that it be given by subcutaneous injection at intervals of 14 to 28 days on an ongoing, open-ended schedule.

Asthma medicines new to the American market include monometasone (Asmanex® Twisthaler®) and levalbuterol (Xopenex®). Monometasone, a daily-use maintenance controller treatment, is a long-acting inhaled corticosteroid. It is FDA-approved for use in children aged 12 years and older and is administered once

Effector cells

Specialized white blood cells (such as macrophages, T cells, B cells, and activated mast cells) that interact and release mediators that create the typical symptoms of an allergic response.

a day as an inhaled dry powder. Levalbuterol is a short-acting β_2 agonist bronchodilator that is derived from albuterol. Although previously available only as a solution for nebulization, levalbuterol is also now manufactured as a hydrofluoroalkane (HFA) metered-dose inhaler. Levalbuterol is believed to have less undesirable effects on heart rate and a slightly longer duration of action compared with albuterol. If a child experiences a "shaky feeling" or tremors when using albuterol, many asthma specialists will substitute levalbuterol.

82. How do I determine what asthma medicines are best for my child?

Effective asthma management includes a true partnership between the treating physician, the patient, and the patient's parents and caregivers. We firmly believe that the selection of which asthma medicines are "best" for a child is the physician's responsibility. You must, of course, as a parent become involved and learn as much as you can about the medicines your child has been prescribed. An effective physician establishes open lines of communication with you and your child such that you should both feel completely at ease sharing any observations and any concerns about medications with the doctor. The first part of our answer to your question is thus: your child's doctor determines which medicines are best for asthma treatment. At that point, your role is twofold. You must make certain that your child is taking the medicines correctly and on schedule. Your second responsibility is to report back to the physician as truthfully and accurately as you can. If you—the parent of a child with asthma—are "doing everything right" and you also believe that your child would benefit from "better" medication, consider obtaining a consultation from an asthma specialist as discussed in Question 88.

The second part of our answer regarding the "best" medicines for your child reviews recent advances in medications for asthma. Allergy plays a significant role as a cause of asthma in many children. For children older than 12 years who have allergic asthma and are not doing well despite a comprehensive medical regimen, a new immunologic treatment is available. Before discussing exactly what this new form of treatment can accomplish, it is necessary to quickly review the immunologic steps that ultimately lead to the appearance of asthma symptoms.

Beginning at the tail end of the process, (1) allergic or asthmatic symptoms develop because several chemical compounds called mediators are released into the circulation from specialized white blood cells (mast cells or basophils) that have been sensitized or primed to react to specific allergens (for example, dog dander, dust mites, pollen grains), and (2) the sensitized mast cell has been coated with specific proteins (IgE antibodies). In traditional immunotherapy (allergy shots), the goal of treatment is to eliminate specific antibodies, for example anti-dog or anti–dust mite antibodies. When this treatment is successful, the child will no longer react allergically to dogs or dust mites. Just imagine: if there was a way to eliminate all or almost all of the circulating IgE and there was no more allergic antibody, theoretically a person would not have an allergic reaction to anything. This novel treatment uses an immunologically modified antibody protein, called a monoclonal antibody, omalizumab (Xolair®). Xolair® has the ability to bind and eliminate circulating IgE. Omalizumab is given through subcutaneous injection every two to four weeks in an open-ended ongoing schedule. For many teenagers and adults with poorly controlled allergic asthma, this new treatment has been highly successful in providing them with a greatly improved quality of life. It must be stressed that this treatment will not cure a child's asthma, but it does provide the physician with a new and effective method of treating appropriately selected patients. If you believe your child is a possible candidate for this treatment, you should discuss this with the allergist or pulmonologist.

A new immunologic treatment is available for children older than twelve years who have allergic asthma.

Xopenex® HFA, a short-acting quick-relief bronchodilator, is now available in a MDI formulation whereas it was previously only manufactured in a liquid form for nebulization. Xopenex® MDI formulation may provide an effective alternative to albuterol in children who feel "jittery" after using albuterol. Xopenex® is an isomer of albuterol (abbreviated l-albuterol) and has a slightly longer duration of action than albuterol, so it is usually dosed at intervals close to eight hours apart. Each person metabolizes medication at a different rate; therefore, you will need to determine how long a single dose of Xopenex controls your child's symptoms.

For years, asthma specialists prescribed the very effective combination of a long-acting inhaled bronchodilator and an anti-inflammatory inhaled corticosteroid. This asthma treatment strategy required using two separate inhalers one after another, immediately back-to-back. An obvious advance was the combination of the two types of asthma medications into one single inhaler device; inhaling one puff from the device would release the two medicines in that one puff. The first combination of a long-acting β_2 bronchodilator and a corticosteroid into one inhaler is the Advair® Diskus®. What makes Advair® novel is that is takes two established asthma drugs, salmeterol (the long-acting β_2 bronchodilator) and fluticasone (the corticosteroid) and delivers them as one puff of medicine. Note that although Advair® is also manufactured as an MDI, only the Advair® DPI known as the Diskus® is approved for use in children ages 4 and up. Advair® Diskus has proved very effective in treating patients with persistent asthma. Early in 2007 another combination preparation called Symbicort® will become available in the United States for treatment of asthma children aged 12 years and older. Symbicort® is in MDI form but is conceptually similar to Advair® as both are inhalers that combine a long-acting β_2 bronchodilator with a corticosteroid. Formoterol is the long-acting β_2 bronchodilator in Symbicort® and the corticosteroid is budesonide. Both budesonide and formoterol have been available as single agents and have been proven to be useful in asthma treatment, and the combined preparation of the two has been available outside the United States for several years.

Recently released mometasone (Asmanex®), a once-daily dry powder inhaled (DPI) corticosteroid preparation, is a welcome addition as a daily use controller medication used for long-term anti-inflammatory management of bronchial asthma. For many years mometasone was used as a topical cream or ointment formulation for eczema and as an intranasal spray for treating allergic rhinitis. The delivery device for the inhaled form, called a Twisthaler®, contains a dry mometasone powder. The drug is currently approved for children aged twelve years and older. The recommendation for once-daily dosing should improve patient adherence in taking the medicine as part of a long-term course of treatment as all other controller corticosteroid medicines require twice-a-day dosing.

Finally, a new once-a-day corticosteroid agent, ciclesonide (Alvesco®), on the horizon, will be marketed as a metered-dose HFA-propelled inhaler. In reports from other countries, the incidence of side effects with ciclesonide, such as oral candidiasis (thrush) and hoarseness, has been extremely low or absent. Although the final reports on growth studies in children have not yet been reported, there should be little or no change in a child's rate of growth because of the low absorption of this drug into the general circulation.

The development of new and better medications is a quest of pharmaceutical companies worldwide.

As indicated earlier, the development of new and better medications is a quest involving the research and development sections of pharmaceutical companies worldwide. From the conception of an idea for a new drug to its availability at your neighborhood pharmacy takes approximately seven to ten years and hundreds of millions of dollars. There is currently ongoing work in the field of asthma and allergy, which optimistically will provide both physicians and patients with highly effective and extremely safe medications that will perhaps one day cure asthma.

83. What is influenza? Why should I or my child get a flu shot (influenza vaccination)?

Influenza is a potentially serious respiratory disease caused by the influenza virus. Influenza viruses are classified as types A, B, or C. Influenza A is further classified into various subtypes. Influenza viruses of the A and B type are responsible for classic influenza illness in humans. The disease is different from the common cold or stomach flu. Influenza is a specific illness, but many people say that they "have the flu" to indicate that they are under the weather or ill in a general way.

Influenza produces widespread sporadic respiratory illness each year during fall and winter in the Northern hemisphere. It has occurred in epidemic or pandemic forms. The symptoms of influenza include the abrupt onset of chills and high fever in the range of 102°F to 103°F. Severe generalized aches and pains, often most intense in the back and legs, accompany the fever. Exhaustion is common, as are headache and loss of appetite. A sensation of pain felt behind the eyeballs is often reported. Respiratory symptoms are initially mild; a scratchy or sore throat can accompany a slight dry cough. The lung symptoms develop later and begin to dominate the picture, with persistent and productive cough an unmistakable feature. Fever can last up to five days in uncomplicated cases. After other symptoms subside, weakness and fatigue may linger for as long as several weeks.

Unfortunately, not all persons who become ill with influenza have an uncomplicated course as described above. Severe, fulminant, or fatal pneumonia can complicate influenza. Influenza is responsible for more than 35,000 deaths and 110,000 hospitalizations each year in the United States alone. Many of the deaths and hospitalizations occur among persons with underlying health conditions that place them at increased risk for complications. Increasing age (50 years or older), very young age (2 years or younger), and pregnancy also place individuals at increased risk for influenza complications. Asthma is also considered a risk factor for potential complications from influenza.

Influenza can now be diagnosed in a few minutes in a doctor's office. If you or your child has symptoms of influenza, the doctor may advise a sample from a nasal wash be tested to detect influenza virus. A person who tests positive for influenza might then be a candidate for immediate treatment with the antiviral medicines oseltamivir (Tamiflu®), which is approved by the U.S. Food and Drug Administration for treating influenza in those aged 1 year and older, or zanamivir (Relenza®), which is approved for older children and adults. Zanamivir is administered through inhalation and may be a less desirable choice in individuals with asthma. Both medicines shorten the time during which influenza can be transmitted to others, and help reduce the severity and duration of illness provided they are taken very early in the course of influenza. Oseltamivir, for example, is effective only if started within forty-eight hours of the onset of influenza symptoms. Taking either medicine later in the course of an established influenza infection does not provide benefit. Oseltamivir is also approved for the prevention (prophylaxis) of influenza in exposed and at-risk adults and in adolescents aged 13 years and older. Neither oseltamivir nor zanamivir is considered a substitute for influenza vaccination.

The single best way to prevent influenza is through vaccination (Table 26). Vaccination against influenza virus causes the body's immune system to manufacture protective antibodies. The antibodies produced in response to successful vaccination will help fight off influenza when and if a person becomes exposed to the virus. Detailed studies of the structure of the influenza virus show that the virus wraps itself in a protective envelope or coat. Influenza is considered a tricky and clever virus because of its ability to change the proteins on its coat. Even subtle changes increase influenza's ability to invade the human body and cause illness. Therefore, the body needs to produce specific yet different protective antibodies directed against different strains of the influenza virus to effectively protect against the development of infection. Antibodies are generally specific and are therefore effective against one strain of influenza virus and unlikely to provide protection against a different strain.

Different strains of influenza circulate each flu season, which is why a person can get the flu two or more years in succession. It is also the reason why each year governmental health agencies advise vaccine manufacturers which specific strains should be included in that year's influenza vaccine. A different influenza vaccine is produced each year. The vaccine available each fall in the United States is effective against three specific influenza strains that health authorities believe will cause most of the serious illness that year. The vaccine you receive in the fall of 2008, for example, can be expected to protect against the common disease-causing strains of influenza circulating in the United States during that winter.

Vaccine

A specialized preparation designed to stimulate the body's immune system to make protective antibodies directed against a specific infectious agent.

Recommendations

195

Table 26   Influenza Vaccination

Vaccination is the best way to prevent illness from influenza. Asthma is an indication for yearly influenza vaccination, beginning at six months of age.

There are two influenza vaccines approved for use in the United States. One is injected into a muscle and the other is sprayed into the nasal passages.

Who should receive the injected influenza vaccine also called the "flu shot"?

Anyone aged 6 months or older with asthma
- Healthy babies and children aged 6 months to 59 months
- All adults beginning at age 50
- Child or teenagers (ages 6 months to 18 years) undergoing long-term aspirin therapy
- Pregnant women who will be in their second or third trimester of pregnancy during influenza season
- Persons aged 6 months old or more with a chronic respiratory (lung) or cardiovascular (heart) condition
- Persons aged 6 months old or more with diabetes, chronic blood, kidney, or immune system disease
- Nursing home and chronic-care facility residents
- Persons likely to transmit influenza to others at high risk for developing influenza complications. The category includes health care providers (doctors, nurses) as well as caregivers, parents, and household contacts of infants and children from birth to age 59 months
- Anyone older than 6 months who (or whose parents) wishes to reduce the likelihood of becoming ill with influenza
- Vaccination may be considered on a case-by-case basis for persons living in dormitories or other crowded conditions (to prevent outbreaks); those providing essential community services (such as firefighters and police); and those at high risk traveling to the Southern hemisphere (April to September), to the tropics, or in organized tourist groups (at any time).

A person who has experienced a significant egg allergy or an allergic reaction to a prior influenza vaccine, or to any influenza vaccine constituent, should not receive the influenza vaccine. A person who has been diagnosed with a disease called Guillain-Barré syndrome should inform their doctor of that diagnosis before receiving an influenza vaccination.

Two different types of influenza vaccines are available for preventing influenza in the United States: an inactivated vaccine and a live, attenuated vaccine (LAIV) (Table 27). The first is an inactivated vaccine. Inactivated means that the vaccine contains a "killed" strain or form of influenza. It is administered by injection into a muscle. The inactivated vaccine is the familiar flu shot that has been in clinical use for many years. The LAIV, on the other hand, contains a weakened strain of influenza and is administered intranasally, by spraying into the nasal passages. The LAIV was first licensed in the United States in 2003. It is manufactured by Wyeth and is named FluMist®. Like the inactivated influenza vaccine, LAIV stimulates the body's production of protective antibodies directed against three strains of influenza currently in circulation. Both vaccines are administered each year, ideally in October or November. LAIV, as of this writing, is only approved for administration to healthy persons between ages 5 and 49 years. It is not currently approved for use in pregnant women or in people who have asthma.

Table 27   Comparison of Available Influenza Vaccines

Inactivated ("killed") Influenza Vaccine	Live, Attenuated ("weakened") Influenza Vaccine
The vaccine is a shot, given by injection into muscle. For children younger than 9 years who are getting the vaccine for the first time, two doses are required.	The vaccine is sprayed into the nostrils. For children younger than 5 to 9 years old who are getting the vaccine for the first time, two doses are required.
The vaccine has been used for many years.	The vaccine was licensed in the United States in 2003 for use in healthy children and adults from 5 to 49 years of age.
The vaccine is recommended for all children aged 6 months and older with asthma.	The vaccine contains a live, attenuated (weakened) form of influenza virus The vaccine is updated each year.
The vaccine contains an inactivated (killed) form of influenza virus and is updated every year.	
The vaccine is best taken in October or November each fall. Vaccination is required yearly.	The inhaled vaccine is currently not advised for pregnant women and people with underlying medical diseases. **It is also currently not recommended for persons with asthma.** It is not recommended for children younger than 5 years or adults older than 50.
Protection begins about fourteen days after vaccination.	
Protection lasts about one year.	
Side effects, if any, are usually mild; soreness at the injection site is the most common. Fever and aches can occur. Call your doctor if you think you are experiencing a more serious side effect.	October or November is the best time for vaccination. It should be repeated yearly.
	Side effects, if any, are usually mild and may include runny nose, congestion, cough, mild fever, aches, fatigue, throat soreness, and, in children, abdominal pain, vomiting, or diarrhea.

Because influenza can be a fatal and devastating illness, especially in certain groups of individuals, vaccination is recommended for those at high risk for developing medical complications from infection with influenza. Medical complications include hospitalization, severe illness manifestations, respiratory failure, and death. All persons with asthma, children and adults alike, are candidates for yearly influenza vaccination. Unvaccinated healthy persons can get sick with influenza and then pass the infection along to others. Only in a few, very specific circumstances is vaccination absolutely contraindicated. Any person who has a significant egg allergy or had an allergic reaction to a prior influenza vaccine or any constituent of the vaccine should not receive the influenza vaccine. Anyone who has been diagnosed with a neurologic condition called Guillain-Barré Syndrome should consult with a physician who is especially knowledgeable about the risks associated with vaccination.

All persons with asthma, children and adults alike, are candidates for yearly influenza vaccination.

In general, influenza vaccination is very safe and effective. You cannot "get the flu" from the inactivated influenza vaccine, nor can the vaccination cause an infection. It is possible, however, to become ill with influenza even if you received the vaccine, because the vaccine does not protect against all strains of influenza. The goal of influenza vaccination is to protect people from becoming severely ill from the virus. Physicians still consider vaccination a success if their patients become ill with a milder form of the flu that slows them down for a few days but does not lead to an exacerbation of their asthma or to hospitalization.

84. I have heard that people can get sick from the influenza vaccine. Will the flu shot make me or my child ill?

It is a myth that influenza vaccine will cause you or your child to become ill with "the flu." You cannot develop influenza from the vaccine. In fact, the exact opposite is true: the vaccine protects its recipients from influenza illness. Vaccination provides protection from severe illness caused by the specific strains of influenza contained in the vaccine. However, just because you or your child will not get influenza from the vaccination does not mean that your child will not get sick at all. If your child was exposed to influenza immediately prior to the vaccination, it is possible that he or she will still get sick, although the vaccine may decrease the severity or duration of the illness. It is also possible that you or your child could become sick from a different germ or virus, or even a strain of influenza other than the one included in the vaccine—but overall, getting the vaccination improves your child's chances of avoiding influenza for that season. (Remember, the vaccine is only applicable to a particular season's strain of influenza; you will need to have your child re-vaccinated the following year.)

The effectiveness of the vaccine in preventing illness is related to your child's general state of health and the specific components contained in the vaccine. Occasionally, some children complain of localized soreness, swelling, or redness at the injection site. With the newer pediatric vaccine formulations, the possibility of developing generalized symptoms such as low-grade fever is quite rare. The "take-home message" regarding influenza vaccination is that any child who has a chronic illness, especially those with lung diseases, should receive yearly immunization against "the flu." The sole exception to this recommendation applies to any child who is allergic to eggs. If your child has an allergic reaction to eggs, discuss the situation with your child's primary care doctor and, if possible, seek a consultation with an allergist.

85. Is it necessary for my child to get the flu vaccine every year?

Yes, unless your child's physician has informed you that vaccination is medically contraindicated. Influenza is a highly contagious disease that returns every year during flu season. Most flu infections occur between November and March, and everyone is at risk for becoming infected with the flu virus.

199

The Centers for Disease Control and Prevention (CDC) publishes yearly recommendations for administering the influenza vaccine. With few exceptions, most people with asthma are appropriate candidates for receiving the vaccine every year, beginning at age 6 months.

With few exceptions, most people with asthma are appropriate candidates for receiving the influenza vaccine every year, beginning at age 6 months.

Certain population groups are at a higher level of risk for developing complications from the flu. These individuals include all children aged 6 to 23 months of age, pregnant women, adults aged 50 years and older, and anyone with chronic health conditions such as asthma, diabetes, anemia as well as lung, heart, and kidney diseases. Additional high-risk groups include children with weakened immune systems secondary to HIV/AIDS, anyone on long-term treatment with corticosteroids, children undergoing chemotherapy or radiation treatment for cancer, and any child between the ages of 6 months and 18 years who requires chronic aspirin therapy.

Currently, two types of influenza vaccine are available, as discussed in Question 83; the traditional form is an inactivated (killed) vaccine administered by intramuscular injection. Since 2003, an attenuated (live, weakened) vaccine has been available that is delivered as a nasal spray. Because many strains of the influenza virus exist and all have a tendency to mutate or change from year to year, the vaccine must be constantly modified. After the vaccine is administered, protective antibodies develop within two to three weeks. The vaccine is effective for approximately one year, which is why it is necessary to be revaccinated annually.

The intranasally administered attenuated flu vaccine is not currently recommended for children who are younger than 5 years or for anyone who has asthma or other chronic heart or lung conditions. Pregnant women and adults older than 49 years should not receive this form of the flu vaccine.

Children may receive the flu vaccine at the same time as their other immunizations. The possibility of developing a severe reaction or symptoms of the flu from the injected (killed)

Recommendations

vaccine is highly unlikely. Any child who has been diagnosed with a severe egg allergy should not be given the influenza vaccine.

All children aged 6 months and older, unless they have a specific contraindication, should receive the flu vaccine every year. Naturally, if you have any questions or concerns regarding any immunization, you should discuss them with your child's physician.

86. Is it dangerous for children who have asthma to take antihistamines?

The answer to the question is no, it is not dangerous to take antihistamines if you have asthma. At one time it was mistakenly believed that the potential drying action of antihistamines on the mucus in the bronchial passageways would aggravate and worsen asthma. Currently available evidence does not support the hypothesis. On the contrary, there is some information to suggest that antihistamines are actually beneficial in children with asthma. We are not recommending that antihistamines be used as a specific treatment for asthma. However, with rare exceptions, children who have both allergic nasal symptoms and asthma should have no problem taking antihistamines. Many physicians do not hesitate to use the antihistamine class of medicine in any child with asthma and allergies who may benefit from their use.

Despite current knowledge regarding the pharmacologic action of antihistamines, package inserts in some of the products still state that patients who have asthma should avoid using them. This is an example of how difficult it is sometimes to change a recommendation once it has appeared in print. We are comfortable prescribing antihistamines for allergy treatment in children with asthma. Antihistamines are generally safe and effective. We also strongly believe that any changes in a child's medical regimen (including the addition of an over-the-counter, non-prescription antihistamine) should be discussed beforehand.

Many physicians feel strongly that any changes in a child's medical regimen should be discussed beforehand.

Kerrin's comment:

My son was prescribed Zyrtec® at the same time he was officially diagnosed with asthma. He takes it every day, along with Singulair®. His asthma symptoms have been well controlled since he started taking these medications, and his allergies have also been manageable.

87. I have heard that some children receive allergy shots to treat their asthma. Should I consider having my child start this treatment? How effective can it be, and what are the risks associated with injection treatment (immunotherapy)?

It has been estimated that 60% to 80% of children with asthma are also allergic. This means that they have an elevated IgE, or allergic antibody level and a positive allergy test (RAST® or skin test) that correlates with their pattern of symptoms. An example might be the child who has a positive test to dog and who wheezes whenever in contact with a dog. As described in the answer to Question 34, the positive test and the child's history are similar to a lock and key that open the door into a room full of symptoms.

Hyposensitization

A decrease, but not total elimination, of a person's ability to develop allergic symptoms to a specific allergen, a result of an immunotherapy regimen.

Asthma symptoms can be triggered by both allergic and nonallergic stimuli. If allergy plays a major role in a child's asthma, then the child may be an appropriate candidate for what is commonly referred to as allergy injection treatment, allergy shots, hyposensitization, or desensitization, or, to be more technically correct, allergen immunotherapy (IT). Immunotherapy involves the subcutaneous injection of specific allergens that have been proven (both by a positive history and by appropriate allergy testing) responsible for causing your child's allergy symptoms. The technique of injecting patients with specific allergens (immunotherapy) has been used as a form of treatment in the clinical practice of allergy for more than eighty years. For practical purposes, allergy injection treatment should be considered a very slow form of immunization. Many months typically pass before any evidence of clinical improvement occurs that can be attributed to the allergy shots. With our current level of understanding and technology, it is difficult (if not impossible) to predict in advance what the ultimate clinical response to immunotherapy will be for each individual child. Immunotherapy has been shown to be effective in treating allergic rhinitis, insect sting allergy, and allergic asthma. However, every child who has asthma is not necessarily an appropriate candidate for allergen immunotherapy.

Immunotherapy is rarely, if ever, indicated for children who are younger than 5 years old. Treatment generally lasts three to five years. Your child's course of treatment will begin with weekly office visits. As the dose of allergen is increased, the interval between visits will progresses from weekly to twice a month, to finally, at the maintenance level, to one visit every three or four weeks. The decision regarding when to discontinue immunotherapy is based on several considerations. Two of the more important points relate to the frequency of your child's symptoms and the requirement for ongoing medication. Your child should ideally be free of symptoms and require minimal or no fast-acting, quick-relief, or inhaled corticosteroid medications for 12 to 18 months before immunotherapy treatment stops.

You should always discuss with your child's physician both the potential benefits and side effects associated with any treatment or medicine prescribed for your child. Regarding immunotherapy, you must understand that your child will be given injections containing the specific allergens that have been responsible for triggering his or her asthma symptoms. For this reason, it is very important that the allergy shots be administered by a physician or other member of the health care team who has experience with this method of treatment.

In general, most patients experience few if any side effects from immunotherapy treatment administered by an experienced practitioner. Among the reactions that may develop, the most common is localized itching and swelling at the injection site. The possibility of a more generalized, systemic allergic response, although far less common, also exists. Such a reaction may present as sneezing, coughing, hives, and wheezing. A severe systemic or anaphylactic reaction could potentially occur during immunotherapy but reactions of such intensity are fortunately rare. Finally, extremely rare case reports of fatal reactions occurring after an allergy injection have appeared in the medical literature. With prompt attention and treatment, adverse reactions to immunotherapy can almost always be immediately controlled on the spot, in the allergist's office, without resorting to the resources of a hospital or an emergency room. For this reason, every single patient undergoing immunotherapy, regardless of how long they have been undergoing immunotherapy (or of how busy their schedule is) must wait in the physician's office for at least twenty minutes after receiving their injections. There should be absolutely no exceptions to this rule. The vast majority of severe reactions will occur within this brief period of observation; a patient who does develops an adverse reaction and who is in the physician's office can be treated quickly and effectively by the physician and the staff.

After the allergist completes your child's evaluation, a comprehensive assessment that reviews the diagnosis and specific treatment recommendations will be discussed with you. Only certain children are considered appropriate candidates for immunotherapy. If your child fulfills the medical criteria established by published guidelines, we recommend you include immunotherapy treatment as a component of your child's comprehensive asthma management program.

Frank's comment:

I was referred to Dr. Feldman way back in the early 1990s by my pediatrician, who recommended I receive allergy shots on a regular basis. They really helped considerably over the years and have overall been a positive treatment for me. Unfortunately, immunotherapy probably isn't for everyone, but for the most part those I know who receive the shots are less likely to suffer severe allergy problems or asthma episodes. If you think your child might benefit from allergy shots, or if the doctor advises it, then perhaps seeing an allergist and receiving a "skin test" might be a great idea. Your child may not express the same fondness for the shots that you might feel, but he or she will thank you in the future.

88. Is it necessary for my daughter to see a specialist, or can her primary care doctor diagnose and treat her asthma?

Most children who have asthma are diagnosed and initially treated by their primary care physician. Of the approximately seven million children with asthma in the United States, only a small percentage are managed by either an allergist or a pulmonologist.

If your child's asthma is mild in severity and well controlled, there may be no reason to see a specialist. The key phrase in the last sentence is *well controlled*. According to the guidelines established by the National Asthma Education and Prevention Program (NAEPP), asthma control has been achieved when your child has no coughing, no difficulty in breathing, no nighttime awakening because of cough or wheeze, no acute asthma episodes, no absences from school or activities, and the parent or caregiver has had no missed time from work. Objectively, your child should have normal or near-normal lung function. If these criteria are fulfilled, your child's asthma is well controlled.

Consultation with a pulmonologist or an allergist is appropriate if the management goals listed above are not achieved. The specialist may make recommendations that he or she believes will improve the ultimate outcome of your child's asthma. Ongoing daily management should be the responsibility of the primary care physician and, depending on its success, return visits to the specialist may or may not be necessary. If problems arise, a discussion between your primary care physician and the specialist may frequently be all that is necessary to control the situation. The combined efforts of parents and physicians working together are an important, if not critical, component of any comprehensive asthma management program and enable your child to achieve the best possible outcome.

PART SEVEN

Specialized Situations

I am pregnant and my six-year-old daughter has asthma. Does that mean my unborn child will have develop asthma?

How can I make sure that my child's school can cope with his allergies and his asthma?

What sports should I encourage for my child with asthma?

More . . .

89. My son has asthma. Is it true that eating dairy products will increase his mucus production and aggravate his cough? Is there a relationship between drinking milk and increased production of mucus?

There is no causal relationship between drinking milk and producing mucus unless you have a true milk allergy. Over time, folklore has developed regarding the role of milk and the production of mucus (Table 28). Milk by itself does not stimulate the production of mucus, and we are not aware of any scientific experiments that have proven that merely drinking milk stimulates mucus-secreting glands to become hyperactive. Because whole milk has more butterfat than 1%, 2%, or skim milk, it may seem like your child produces more mucus; however, this is merely a perception and not a fact.

Table 28   Asthma Myths and Falsehoods

Wheezing is a fact of life for a child with asthma.
Asthma is contagious; a child can pass it to a classmate, friend, or relative.
Asthma is all in the mind and only emotionally needy or disturbed children have asthma.
Children with asthma should not participate in team sports.
Children with asthma should be permanently excused from physical education class.
Using inhaler medicines regularly will cause psychological dependency and "addiction" to asthma medicines.
It is better to use an inhaler only when a child has symptoms than to use one to prevent symptoms.
Using inhaled corticosteroid medication stunts children's growth.
Milk causes mucus production and should be avoided by children with asthma.
Moving to a hot, dry climate will cure asthma.
Asthma is a purely psychological disease.
Mothers with asthma should never breastfeed.

A child diagnosed with asthma who never wheezes doesn't have asthma.

Children will eventually outgrow their asthma and be cured by the time they become adults.

Children who are truly allergic to milk will produce more mucus if they are exposed to dairy products. During an allergic reaction to milk, mucus-secreting glands are stimulated to produce significantly greater amounts of mucus that may appear to be thicker than normal.

Some children may be uncomfortable drinking whole milk during a respiratory tract infection or when experiencing symptoms of asthma. If that has been your child's experience, you can temporarily discontinue dairy products or switch to either skim or 1% milk until the acute symptoms disappear. Skim milk has all the nutritional benefits of whole milk; the only difference is the absence of the butterfat.

90. Can acupuncture or other alternative treatments cure my child's asthma?

Objective reviews of published studies that use acupuncture to treat bronchial asthma are inconclusive. The available data have failed to clearly show either benefit or harm. The consensus among American experts is that additional high-quality research must be performed before recommendations can be made regarding the effectiveness of alternative therapeutic approaches to asthma. It is important to remember that, as of 2007, medical science has no absolute method of curing asthma (see Question 22). Asthma can, however, be very effectively controlled, permitting children and adults with this disease to lead full, active lives. Asthma specialists practicing in the United States believe that the use of anti-asthma medications plays a crucial role in maintaining optimal control of children's asthma symptoms and that they are the foundation of a comprehensive asthma management program.

It is important for children with asthma and their parents to learn as much as possible about the disease. The knowledge combined with ongoing consultation with the treating physician will help patients and their families develop the necessary self-management skills that are an essential component of successful asthma care. Exercise and adherence to a healthy lifestyle are as important as measuring peak flows and using inhaler medicines. The National Institutes of Health (NIH) has committed to addressing "approaches to health care that are outside the realm of conventional medicine as practiced in the United States." To that end, Congress in 1998 established the National Center for Complementary and Alternative Medicine (NCCAM). The NCCAM is one of twenty-seven institutes and centers that make up the NIH. The NIH is one of eight agencies under the Public Health Service in the Department of Health and Human Services. The NCCAM is "dedicated to exploring complementary and alternative healing practices in the context of rigorous science, training complementary and alternative medicine (CAM) researchers, and disseminating authoritative information to the public and professionals." It is located in Bethesda, Maryland on the NIH complex and maintains a comprehensive and informative Web site (http:/www.nccam.nih.gov/) where you can obtain reliable information on alternative and complementary treatments for asthma and various other illnesses.

The term complementary medicine refers to treatments that supplement or complement traditional medical treatments. Alternative medical treatments, on the other hand, have the goal of completely replacing traditional medical therapies with alternatives. Alternative treatments essentially reject the approach to asthma we recommend. Complementary asthma therapies are designed to be used alongside the asthma treatments included in this book. Some patients with asthma we care for have explored yoga, swimming therapy, meditation, traditional Chinese medicine (including herbs), acupuncture, breathing exercises, and homeopathic remedies while adhering to their asthma treatment plans. If you have questions about any of these complementary treatment methods, we recommend you begin gathering information by first speaking to the members of the medical team who are directly involved in your child's care.

91. I am pregnant and my 6-year-old daughter has asthma. Does this mean that my second child will develop asthma?

Because your 6-year-old daughter has asthma, there is a statistically increased risk that your second child will also have asthma. Understand that although asthma tends to run in families, it is not certain that if one child has this condition, your other children will also. Although our knowledge of genetics is increasing significantly year by year, we currently do not have the ability to manipulate individual genes to eliminate or modify a child's potential to develop a specific disease, such as asthma.

In addition to a genetic predisposition to developing asthma, environmental factors play a definite role in influencing who may be at risk for developing this condition. There are children without any family history of asthma or allergy who nevertheless develop recurring chest symptoms of cough and wheeze. We are becoming more knowledgeable about environmental factors and their relationship to asthma, and what can be done to decrease the effect of these situations.

92. Is there anything I can do during pregnancy to prevent my unborn child from developing asthma?

No specific intervention exists that will modify a child's probability of developing asthma. If you already have one child with allergy symptoms or asthma, however, there are a few measures you can take during your pregnancy that may possibly modify your unborn child's potential for developing asthma. If you are a smoker, you must quit immediately. Children born of mothers who smoke during their pregnancy have an increased incidence of wheezing in infancy. If you do not smoke, you should also avoid exposure to second-hand smoke. Continue to maintain the environmental control measures in your home that were recommended for your first child. When planning meals, limit your intake of the more highly allergenic foods (such as tree nuts, peanuts, shellfish, eggs, and dairy products) as their absence in the maternal diet seems to delay the onset of allergy symptoms in a young child. Avoiding alcoholic beverages is recommended during pregnancy. Consider breastfeeding your child for at least the first three, and preferably six, months of their life. Breast milk has been shown to support and stimulate the development of your child's immune system. Finally, prenatal care beginning as early as possible in your pregnancy is critical in providing your newborn child with the best possible health at birth.

For some children, the development of allergy or asthma is inevitable despite all your best efforts at following experts' recommendations. Appropriate pediatric care coupled with early recognition and treatment of asthma symptoms makes a significant difference in the ultimate outcome of your child's asthma. Discuss the situation and any concerns you may have with your child's allergist or pulmonologist to see if they have additional, more individualized recommendations for you.

93. I have asthma and I am pregnant. Is it safe to use asthma medicines during my pregnancy? Should I stop taking my asthma medications?

Discussions concerning pregnancy, asthma, and medicine can be complicated. As a rule of thumb, one third of pregnant women with asthma will experience an improvement of their asthma in pregnancy, one third will have a worsening of their symptoms, and one third's asthma will be unaffected by the pregnancy. The ideal pregnancy from a medication standpoint would be one in which no medicine was required. It would be wonderful, but unrealistic, to suggest that a woman who has asthma could complete her pregnancy without requiring any anti-asthma medication. How can physicians minimize medication risks for both the mother and her unborn child?

As you might well imagine, this dilemma has been the topic of discussion among specialists in the fields of pharmacology, obstetrics, neonatology, pulmonology, and allergy. A great deal of time, money, and effort has been spent in attempting to resolve this very difficult-to-answer question. The current recommendations, which are always subject to revision, represent a consensus based on the most reliable scientific information currently available.

The most recent comprehensive report regarding the management of asthma during pregnancy was published in 2004. The recommendations of the National Asthma Education and Prevention Program (NAEPP) are based on a detailed review of studies that appeared in the medical literature from 1993 until 2003. There is widespread agreement that aggressive treatment of asthma symptoms is of primary importance in allowing the pregnancy to proceed to term and to achieve the most favorable outcome for both mother and child.

Drug safety in pregnancy is assessed for each medication by the U.S. Food and Drug Administration (see Question 94). For mild intermittent asthma symptoms, the preferred short-acting bronchodilator is albuterol. To control symptoms labeled persistent, an inhaled corticosteroid is the preferred medication. Within this class, the drug that has been involved in most studies is budesonide. However, if a woman has been using another inhaled steroid, the recommendation is to continue using the same medication throughout the pregnancy. If there is need for a long-acting bronchodilator, salmeterol would be the first choice, primarily because it has been used in this country longer than formoterol.

Oral (systemic) corticosteroids have been perscribed for women who are pregnant; if their use is absolutely necessary, they should be administered, albeit with great care. Oral corticosteroids have been associated with preeclampsia in some pregnant women, as well as with early-delivery and low birth weight infants. The volume of data that is currently available is not adequate to permit an absolute statement about the short-term use of systemic steroids in women who are pregnant. Oral steroid use should therefore be limited to women who are experiencing severe asthma during their pregnancy. Drugs such as theophylline, cromolyn, and leukotriene modifiers are listed as alternative, but not preferred, treatments for asthma during pregnancy.

Many women with asthma frequently have allergic rhinitis and sinusitis. These conditions can be treated during pregnancy with intranasal steroids and the second-generation antihistamines, loratadine and cetirizine. During the first trimester of pregnancy, pseudoephedrine should be avoided. Currently, data regarding the use of montelukast to treat pregnant women with allergic rhinitis are insufficient to make a recommendation.

If you are planning to become pregnant, you should consult both your obstetrician and your allergist or pulmonologist about how to manage your asthma while you are pregnant. If you become pregnant unexpectedly, consult with your physicians early in your pregnancy and establish a treatment plan before problems develop. Under all circumstances, it is extremely important for pregnant women to treat symptoms of asthma early and aggressively.

At the opposite end of the question of drug safety lies the question of what happens if you take no asthma medications. The single biggest risk to a pregnancy in a woman with asthma is poor asthma control. Uncontrolled asthma is very harmful

Sinusitis

An inflammation of the lining of sinuses caused most commonly by either infection (viral or bacterial sinusitis) or allergy (allergic sinusitis).

It is extremely important for pregnant women to treat symptoms of asthma early and aggressively.

to the developing baby and can result in devastating complications for both mother and child. Possible complications of
poorly controlled asthma include elevated blood pressure, preeclampsia, eclampsia, and preterm labor for the mother. The
child may be born prematurely, develop intrauterine growth
retardation, and have low birth weight at delivery, along with
increased perinatal morbidity and mortality. Inadequate control of the mother's asthma leads to a reduced oxygen supply
to the developing baby (maternal hypoxia) and a decreased
blood supply to the womb. These are serious and potentially
life-threatening situations for both mother and child; the
risks of using various medications are usually considerably
lower. All medical specialists agree that they should treat their
pregnant patients with asthma medicines that are not only
highly effective but also as safe as possible for both mother
and baby. One fact cannot be emphasized strongly enough:
uncontrolled or inadequately treated asthma represents a far
greater potential danger to both the pregnant woman and her
developing fetus than any possible risk associated with taking
asthma medicine.

94. What are the potential risks of using asthma medications with respect to my unborn child?

The U.S. Food and Drug Administration (FDA) is the governmental agency responsible for approving all prescription
medications in the United States. This group has established
a classification related to the use of drugs in pregnancy. Medicines have been divided into the following classifications: A,
B, C, D, and X (Table 29). No medications are labeled class A
for use in pregnancy, because this designation would indicate
that studies were performed with women who were pregnant
at the time the drug was administered and no such studies
exist. Therefore, the safest medicines are found in the category B classification, which is based on anecdotal reporting

*Uncontrolled
or inadequately
treated asthma
represents a
far greater
potential
danger to both
a pregnant
woman and
her developing
fetus than any
possible risk
associated with
taking asthma
medicine.*

Specialized Situations

involving long-term use in pregnant women and extensive studies involving pregnant laboratory animals that produced no evidence of harmful side effects. A category C designation indicates that the drug has been responsible for some adverse effect on the fetus in animal studies. Drugs in this category may perhaps carry an increased potential developmental risk to the fetus, but they are still considered reasonably safe for use in pregnant women in part because the dose of medicine used in these animal studies is far, far greater than would ever be given to a pregnant woman. The decision to use a medication in this risk category (C) must be determined on a case-by-case basis. A situation must exist in which the potential risk for not using the medication outweighs the lesser risk associated with taking the drug. The overriding consideration in treating acute asthma symptoms in pregnant women must be to control the symptoms as rapidly and effectively as possible.

Table 29   The FDA's Classification of Medicines in Pregnancy

Category	Description
Category A	Adequate and well-controlled studies in pregnant women have not shown an increased risk for fetal abnormalities. *Controlled studies show no risk.*
Category B	Animal studies have revealed no evidence of harm to the fetus, but there are no adequate and well-controlled studies in pregnant women. Or... Studies in animals have shown an adverse effect on the animal fetus but adequate and well-controlled studies in pregnant women have failed to demonstrate a risk to the human fetus. *No evidence of risk in humans.*
Category C	Studies in animals have shown an adverse effect on the animal fetus, and there are no adequate and well-controlled studies in pregnant women to assess risk to the human fetus. Or... No animal studies of the medicine have been performed, and there are no adequate and well-controlled studies in pregnant women to assess risk to the human fetus. *Risk cannot be ruled out.*

Category	Description
Category D	Studies, both adequate and well-controlled, or observational, have demonstrated a risk to the fetus. *Benefits of therapy with this category of medicine in pregnancy may outweigh the potential risk to the fetus.* *Positive evidence of risk.*
Category X	Studies, adequate and well-controlled, or observational, in animals or humans have demonstrated positive evidence of *fetal abnormalities. The use of the medicine is contraindicated in women who are pregnant or who may become pregnant.* *Contraindicated in pregnancy.*

Most medicines used in asthma treatment fall into category C, and several are classified in category B. All short-acting β_2 agonist quick-relief inhaled bronchodilator medications, for example, are classified as category C, even though they have been used for more than two decades and are widely viewed as very safe by the medical profession. They have not been shown to have adverse effects on the course of pregnancy and have not been shown to be harmful to the human fetus. All long-acting β_2 agonist inhaled bronchodilators are also category C medicines. The C classification for the β_2 agonist group of inhalers reflects the absence of studies in pregnant women (as opposed to pregnant animals!). One inhaled corticosteroid preparation, Pulmicort® (budesonide), is category B; all other inhaled steroids are, as of this writing, labeled category C. The long-term inhaled controller medicines Intal® (cromolyn) and Tilade® (nedocromil) are category B, as are the leukotriene modifier tablets Singulair® (montelukast sodium) and Accolade® (zafirlukast). The new IgE blocker Xolair® (omalizumab) carries a category B rating. The theophylline medicines are all category C drugs.

Because both uncontrolled and poorly controlled asthma in the mother have such serious consequences for both her and her unborn child (see Question 93), the guiding principle of treating asthma in pregnancy is to achieve optimal asthma control even if daily medication is required. It is crucial to normalize maternal lung function and ensure that the mother is not experiencing any symptoms of asthma. Pulmonologists believe that any medicine that is required for optimal asthma treatment should be administered to a pregnant woman. For example, steroid bursts are used in pregnancy just as they are when a woman is not pregnant. As a rule of thumb, category B medicines would be used first, with any required medicines that may fall into the C category (or even D) added if necessary to achieve good asthma control.

The guiding principle of treating asthma in pregnancy is to achieve optimal asthma control even if daily medication is required.

If you are pregnant and have any questions or any concerns about the safety of the medicines you have been prescribed, you should consult with your treating physicians. Both your obstetrician and your asthma doctor have the expertise to counsel you and give advice that is best for you. Under no circumstances should you discontinue your prescribed asthma regimen or not follow the treatment plans recommended by your doctor.

95. How can I help my son's school staff learn about and can cope with his allergies and/ or asthma, and know how to deal with an emergency?

The best way to make sure that your son's school is in a position to handle his asthma is to first teach him about his asthma and his allergic condition—to the extent that this is possible depending on his age—and then establish good communication with his teachers and school nurse. Even though childhood asthma is very common, it is good idea to make sure that the school staff knows about your son's asthma and allergies. You should meet with your child's teacher and possibly the nurse (if there is one) early in the school year to discuss your child's medical history. It would be appropriate to have a list of (1) the daily medications that your child takes and (2) the drugs that may have to be administered to treat an acute situation, such as bronchodilator MDIs (albuterol) for asthma or epinephrine (Epi-Pen®, Twinject®) for a severe allergy reaction. Your son's physician may help by preparing a school asthma action plan, as discussed in Question 71. You should in addition make sure that any forms required by the school to allow medication administration are competed before the term begins.

You should familiarize yourself with the school district's policies (if any) regarding the use of medication in the school setting. For example, some schools allow students to carry their bronchodilator inhaler with them at all times, whereas others require that it be left in the school nurse's office. The former is obviously more desirable than the latter. We insist that our patients carry their inhaled bronchodilator with them throughout the school day. The NAEPP and other authorities agree that students with asthma should be allowed to carry their asthma medicine (especially the quick-relief inhaler) for self-administration as required during the school day (with prior parental and physician okay of course!). Review any concerns that you may have with your child's doctor at the beginning of the school year; a good time might be when the physician fills out the required pre-enrollment health forms. The school should be given a written copy of the treatment plan and your son's medication list. Make sure that your son learns when and how to use his fast-acting quick-relief inhaler. He should also, if he is old enough, learn the correct technique for using an MDI without a spacer even though he usually would use an MDI and spacer combination, just to be "on the safe side." You can also check several very useful, patient-centered asthma Internet sites for additional pointers (see the Appendix).

Kerrin's comment:

The day care where my son goes has many people who are familiar with how to work the nebulizer. Because allergies and asthma are so prevalent these days, it's not difficult to find people knowledgeable about the condition and treatment. Whenever he has a cold,

Epinephrine

A naturally occurring hormone produced by the human adrenal glands. A synthetic form (adrenaline) is used to treat severe allergic reactions (anaphylaxis) and life-threatening asthma.

Specialized Situations

You should familiarize yourself with your child's school's policy (if any) regarding asthma in general and inhaler use in particular.

we send the nebulizer and vials of albuterol in to school with him, and one of the teachers administers a treatment before he goes down for a nap and later in the afternoon before I pick him up. This way he is able to get the four treatments per day that his doctor recommends during the times when he is at the greatest risk for having his asthma symptoms triggered.

Frank's comment:

Since children probably spend approximately 60% of the day at school, it is vital that school personnel be aware of any student's asthma and are able to handle any problems. The school nurse is most likely a good place to start. Make sure that he/she is supplied with the necessary equipment to provide for your child's needs (bronchodilator MDI, nebulizer, and medicine). Introducing your son/daughter to the school health care provider is a good idea, since this will make them more comfortable if they should need to go to the nurse. Keeping in touch with the nurse might be a good idea as well. Double check the school standards and policies to make sure all requirements regarding medication use in school are met. Most importantly, make sure your son/daughter is well instructed on how to use their own medication.

96. Our 10-year-old daughter, who has asthma, wants to go to sleep-away camp next summer. Should she go to a regular camp or one exclusively for children who have asthma?

As with many things in life, the answer to this question is, it depends. It depends on (1) the severity of your daughter's asthma symptoms and her level of asthma control on treatment, (2) how frequently she has chest discomfort (if any) that limits her ability to participate in athletics, and (3) possibly most importantly, how well your daughter copes both practically and emotionally with her asthma symptoms.

Like a pendulum, our feelings about camps that are limited to children with a specific medical condition swing back and forth. For a child who has recently been diagnosed with asthma, being in an environment where all the children have this condition can be very positive. Your child will learn that she is not the only one who has to live with asthma. More importantly, the constructive examples of good self-management skills exhibited by the other, more knowledgeable children with asthma will go a long way toward improving your daughter's appreciation of the fact that she can control her symptoms, thereby increasing her self-image.

In the unique environment that an asthma camp provides, your child will not only have a good social experience but, equally importantly, will become more confident in her ability to deal with a potential pattern of recurring symptoms. Children who go to an asthma camp will become more informed about their disease and therefore will be more effective in taking an active role in self-management. Depending on their age, children will learn how and when to take their medications and become accustomed to the routine of a regular dosing schedule. The time spent at camp can provide an intensive educational experience, which is critical for the development of appropriate asthma self-management skills.

The increased knowledge that comes from attending an asthma camp and the self-confidence your child will develop from realizing that she can control the disease most of the time (rather than the other way around) makes it an invaluable experience. Many children realize, and some for the first time, that they can participate in almost all sports activities. Through age-appropriate teaching, campers will learn why they need to take their medicines. As a direct result of the time spent at camp, most children will have fewer unscheduled asthma visits to their pediatrician and the emergency room upon their return.

Naturally, the ultimate goal for any child with a chronic medical condition is for them to function as near to normal, to their potential and to their dreams, as possible. Children who have asthma can accomplish this goal within the framework of an appropriate, comprehensive asthma management plan. Asthma should not compromise your child's ability to perform well at school, on the athletic field, or at home. Time spent at an asthma camp can provide your child with the self-management tools to help make this happen. However, like so many other things, rarely "does one size fit all," and therefore not every child who has asthma must or should only go to an asthma-oriented camp. For some children, a potential problem with going to an asthma camp is that too much attention is focused on the disease and not enough on the other social, educational, and athletic aspects of a camp experience. Many children with asthma have had fantastic camp experiences at regular summer camps. Each child's situation is different; deciding which type of camp will provide the best experience for a particular child is an individual's choice.

You can find a list of asthma camps on the Internet at: *www.asthmacamps.org*.

97. Will my child's weight affect his asthma?

A suspected relationship between obesity and asthma continues to stimulate medical interest. Physicians and the general public have long suspected a possible cause-and-effect relationship between obesity and asthma. The incidence of both obesity and asthma is increasing in western societies. Several population studies have shown an association between being overweight and the likelihood of having asthma. However, the exact relationship between the two conditions remains controversial.

Does asthma cause obesity? Does obesity cause asthma? Could there be a common underlying factor that contributes to the development of both conditions? One traditional explanation

Obesity

The condition of being significantly overweight or obese. A person is obese if they weigh more than 30% above their ideal body weight for their given age, height, and gender. Another definition of obesity involves computation of the BMI. An overweight adult has a BMI of between 25 and 30, whereas an obese adult has a BMI of 30 or greater.

maintains that asthma, particularly if it is not well managed, leads to a more sedentary lifestyle. This lack of physical activity, coupled with the increased appetite of children in their preteen and adolescent years, eventually leads to obesity. Many children with asthma do not exercise, either because of a mistaken belief that athletic activity is harmful in asthma or because their asthma is not well controlled and flares with exercise. An alternative concept suggests that obesity develops first and that the child's excessive weight somehow leads to functional changes in the lungs and the typical pattern of symptoms that is recognized as asthma. Both theories have merits, but each one has conceptual gaps; neither satisfactorily explains why the incidence of asthma does not affect men and women equally, for example. A third, more current idea, which has intriguing supporting data from laboratory animals, attempts to explore the influences of chromosomal changes and hormonal factors, which conceivably could stimulate the simultaneous development of both conditions.

Several population studies have shown an association between being overweight and the likelihood of having asthma.

A key to better understanding the obesity–asthma link may come from the study of girls and boys in puberty and adolescence. More than one thousand children born between May 1980 and January 1984 were at birth entered in the ambitious and ongoing Tucson Children's Respiratory Study. Nearly thirteen hundred babies were enrolled into the study, and they have been followed up and reassessed at regular intervals for more than twenty years by Dr. Fernando Martinez and his team. The prospective study was designed to observe patterns of respiratory health and illness during childhood, adolescence, and early adult life. In particular, the development of asthma was carefully evaluated. In 2001, Dr. Martinez and his coworkers reported that girls who became overweight or obese between the ages of 6 and 11 years of age had an increased risk for developing new asthma symptoms during early adolescence. They found that girls, but not boys, who became overweight between 6 and 11 years of age were 5.5 to 7 times more likely to develop new asthma symptoms at

Puberty

The time during which sexual maturation begins. Also refers to the time when reproductive organs develop to allow reproduction.

Specialized Situations

ages 11 and 13 compared with the girls who did not become overweight or obese at ages 6 and 11 years. Boys who became significantly overweight at those same ages did not exhibit an increased risk for developing asthma or asthma-like symptoms between the ages of 6 and 11 years of age. The strongest association between overweight status and asthma risk was therefore seen in females who underwent puberty before the age of 11 years.

Being overweight is associated with an earlier onset of puberty. Could a common factor lead to overweight status in girls, followed by early puberty and then the development of asthma? The findings are especially interesting because it has long been observed that new cases of asthma in females are especially common in the adolescent years. Furthermore, the increased male-to-female (2:1) ratio of asthma documented in young, school-aged children reverses, so that more girls than boys have asthma as they become adults. A possible role for female hormones has long been suspected and data from the Tucson Children's Respiratory Study support, this theory and provide opportunities for ongoing research.

Apart from the association between obesity and the increased risk for asthma, being overweight is medically undesirable. Even patients with very well-controlled asthma symptoms often report that their breathing is much easier when they maintain a comfortable weight; they feel more limber and less achy, and describe greater endurance. It makes sense that if you carry excess weight on your frame, it literally feels as though you are working harder to transport those additional pounds as you walk around.

How can you tell if you or your child is obese? An obese adult is, by definition, a person who weighs 30% or more above their predicted or ideal body weight. Evaluation of appropriate weight in children is based on the determination of a measurement called the body mass index (BMI). BMI is a measure that can also be used in adults. Assessment of BMI requires accurate measurement of height and weight, usually in meters and kilograms. The BMI is the weight (in kilograms) divided by the square of the height (in meters). You can obtain a table of predicted BMI for any age to compare your child's BMI to the standard. A child with a BMI greater or equal to the 95th percentile for their age is considered obese. If you prefer not to do the math, there are several clever Web sites that ask you to enter data such as your weight, height, and age, and then calculate ideal body weight and BMI for you. Simply go to your preferred search engine, and type a phrase such as "ideal body weight calculator" or "BMI computation" to navigate among the different sites. If you're concerned about your child's weight—whether you think your child is underweight or overweight—talk to his or her pediatrician, who has a better understanding of what an appropriate weight for a child of that age and body type should be.

98. What sports should be encouraged for children with asthma?

We encourage a child to participate in any sport that he or she is interested in. Regular exercise is important for health, and sports should play a role in any child's life, regardless of whether they are diagnosed with asthma or not. When a patient wants to play a team sport or participate in a particular athletic activity, physicians should help them realize their goal.

Some types of exercise are especially advisable in the setting of asthma, whereas others have a greater potential to trigger exercise-induced bronchospasm (EIB) (see Questions 66 and 67). In the latter category, distance running or cross-country skiing, for example, can cause symptoms of cough, breathlessness, or wheezing. Distance running, cycling, and cross-country skiing involve very good aerobic conditioning, but the activity is steady, without breaks or interruption, and takes place in the outdoor environment with exposure to temperature variation, aeroallergens, and sometimes atmospheric

Sports should play a role in any child's life, regardless of whether he or she is diagnosed with asthma or not.

Specialized Situations

pollutants. Athletic activities that incorporate breaks in the intensity of exertion, including competitive sports such as tennis, baseball, golf, volleyball, and lacrosse, are less likely to cause asthma symptoms because they allow time to "catch your breath." Exercise and sports should be encouraged for all asthma patients.

For the majority of children who have asthma, there should be no limitation in their ability to participate in any sport. The use of a short-acting bronchodilator, such as albuterol, inhaled 20 to 30 minutes before active participation may be indicated for a child with asthma and exercise-induced bronchospasm, and should provide sufficient protection to permit them to enjoy their sport.

Even children with well-controlled asthma may experience an asthma exacerbation from time to time, as discussed in Question 32. Part of the treatment of the exacerbation will likely include a temporary "break" from strenuous physical activity, including sports and athletic competitions. When control of asthma is re-established, then your child should be able to resume his or her favorite sports!

Parents sometimes ask what sport may be best for their child with asthma. Swimming is an excellent form of exercise for any age child. The warm, humid air in an indoor swimming pool is especially gentle to asthmatic lungs and unlikely to trigger symptoms. Swimming is also outstanding aerobic exercise. It develops muscle groups symmetrically and helps develop a healthy awareness of breathing while increasing a person's overall fitness and well-being. Because swimming is not a contact sport, musculoskeletal injuries are rare. Swimming is a form of exercise that you can enjoy your entire life. Be aware, however, that swimming in a cold atmosphere, in water that is too cold, or in a heavily chlorinated pool can trigger asthma. Ozone treatment and disinfection of swimming pools has been practiced in Europe for more than fifty years, and is slowly being introduced and accepted in the United States. Swimming pools disinfected primarily with ozone have enhanced water clarity and greatly reduced chemical odors. The pool water is purer and far less irritating to skin, eyes, and lungs. If you live in an area with a choice of pools to swim in, you may want to research whether any of the pools are disinfected with ozone. For instance, the first commercial indoor pool in New York that was primarily disinfected by ozone is located in New York City, at the 92nd Street Y in Manhattan.

Sports that have been associated with greater EIB include track, cross-county running, soccer, field hockey, distance swimming, ice hockey, and cross-country skiing. You will notice that they all involve endurance high-ventilation activity, and several are also winter sports. Sports that tend to cause lesser EIB are golf, baseball, softball, bowling, football, volleyball, and gymnastics. In conclusion, well-controlled asthma is no barrier to fitness and sport. Let your child decide which sport he or she likes best.

99. How should I pack my daughter's asthma medicine when we are traveling by air?

Always, always, always place asthma medicine in a carry-on bag when you travel by air. One obvious reason is that your child may need to use her inhaled asthma medicine during the flight or at the airport, and you will want to have it handy. You should not pack medicine in your checked luggage. Checked suitcases are stored in the hold of the aircraft, which is neither heated nor pressurized to the same standards as the passenger cabin. Most medicine needs to be kept at or close to room temperature. Remember also that checked suitcases are frequently delayed or lost, unlike a bag you keep in your possession. Imagine what a vacation would be like if your daughter's medicine arrived three days after you did!

Before you travel, make sure that you have enough of your daughter's prescription asthma and allergy medicines to last the duration of your trip. You should bring all the usual maintenance asthma drugs and any quick-relief inhalers to use on an as-needed basis. You should also travel with epinephrine auto-injectors if your child has experienced anaphylaxis from severe allergy. Auto-injectors are permitted in carry-on luggage but must be in their original packaging, with the pharmacy's dispensing label affixed. As of this writing, the Transportation Security Administration (TSA) requests that you "declare" the epinephrine by notifying the security screeners at the security checkpoint that you are carrying auto-injectors for your child's medical condition. You are not required to travel with a letter from your child's physician confirming the medical necessity of traveling with auto-injectors, but many physicians will gladly write you such a letter if you ask them to. You can obtain the latest information on traveling by air with medicines at the TSA Website (www.tsa.gov), and in particular at: http://www.tsa.gov/travelers/airtravel/specialneeds/. Nebulizers are permitted in carry-on bags; any batteries must be disconnected, and the machine cannot be used in flight.

Before traveling, parents should make sure they have enough of their child's prescription asthma and allergy medicines to last the duration of the trip.

The patient's name on any prescription's label must match the passenger's identification papers. If you are traveling outside of the United States, it is a good idea to check in with your physician ahead of time to see if you should bring along any additional medicines, such as corticosteroids, antibiotics, or epinephrine. Even though communication by phone anywhere in the world is now easily achieved, obtaining a prescription medication on a moment's notice in a country far from your doctor can become very complicated.

100. Where can I go from here for additional information on my child's asthma?

The Appendix that follows provides several resources for parents with children who have asthma, older children who have asthma, and others interested in this topic. It includes books, government publications, agency contact information, and Internet sites. When using the Internet, remember that not all information you find there is accurate, scientific, or up to date. In the United States and most other parts of the world, URLs that have an ".edu," ".gov," or ".org" at the end of their address are noncommercial sites, whereas those that end in ".com" or ".co" are commercial sites. You need to be careful about your use of Internet information. If in doubt, always speak with your physician for answers to any of your questions.

Specialized Situations

Appendix

Asthma Resources

Asthma resources include books, pamphlets, educational materials, Web sites, and, of course, your physician. Remember that if you have a specific clinical question or concern about your child's asthma or how to specifically treat your child's asthma, you should seek personalized advice from your child's physician.

Books

Books for Children and Young People:

Several very good books on the topic of asthma for children are currently out of print. They may, however, be available from lending libraries and used booksellers.

All About Asthma by William Ostrow, Vivian Ostrow, and Blanche Sims. A. Whitman, 1989. ISBN 0-8075-0275-8.

Asthma by Alvin Silverstein, Virginia B. Silverstein, and Laura Silverstein-Nunn. Scholastic Library Publishing, 2001. ISBN 0-5311-2048-1.

Breathe Easy: Young People's Guide to Asthma by Jonathan H. Weiss and Michael Chesworth. American Psychological Association, 2003. ISBN 1-5579-8956-7.

Hometown Hero: Featuring Scott Whittaker by Barbara Aiello, Jeffrey Shulman, and Loel Barr. Millbrook Press, 1991. ISBN 0-9414-7704-5.

Luke Has Asthma, Too by Allison Rogers and Michael Middleton. Waterfront Books, 1988. ISBN 0-9145-2506-9.

Thin Air by David Getz. Henry Holt & Company, 1990. ISBN 0-8050-1372-2.

Books on Asthma for Parents and Teens:

A Parent's Guide to Asthma: How You Can Help Your Child Control Asthma at Home, School and Play by Nancy Sander. Plume, 1994. ISBN 0-4522-7216-5.

American Academy of Pediatrics Guide to Your Child's Asthma and Allergies: Breathing Easy and Bringing up Healthy, Active Children by Michael J. Welch (editor). Random House, 2000. ISBN 0-6797-6982-X.

Breathe Easy!: A Teen's Guide to Allergies and Asthma by Jean Ford. Mason Crest Publishers, 2004. ISBN 1-5908-4842-X.

The Asthma and Allergy Action Plan for Kids: A Complete Program to Help Your Child Live a Full and Active Life by Allen J. Dozor and Kate Kelly. Simon & Schuster Adult Publishing Group, 2004. ISBN 0-7432-3577-0.

The Children's Hospital of Philadelphia Guide to Asthma: How to Help Your Child Live a Healthier Life by Children's Hospital of Philadelphia Staff, Nicholas A. Pawlowski (editor) and Tyra Bryant-Stevens (editor). John Wiley & Sons, Inc., 2004. ISBN 0-4714-4116-3.

The Complete Kid's Allergy and Asthma Guide: Allergy and Asthma Information for Children of All Ages by Milton Gold (editor). Robert Rose Inc., 2003. ISBN 0-7788-0079-2.

Books on Asthma:

African Americans' Guide to Managing Asthma by Leroy M Graham. Simon & Schuster Adult Publishing Group, 2004. ISBN 0-7434-6645-4.

Asthma for Dummies by William E. Berger. John Wiley & Sons, Inc., 2004. ISBN 0-7645-4233-8.

The Harvard Medical School Guide to Taking Control of Asthma by Christopher H. Fanta, Kenan Haver, Lynda Cristiano, with Nancy Waring. Simon & Schuster Trade, 2003. ISBN 0-7432-2487-7.

What To Do When the Doctor Says It's Asthma by Paul Hannaway. Rockport Publishers, 2004. ISBN 1-5923-3104-1.

Organizations

American Academy of Allergy, Asthma and Immunology (AAAAI)
611 East Wells Street, Milwaukee, WI 53202
1-800-822-2762
www.aaaai.org
The AAAAI is the largest professional medical specialty organization in
the United States representing professionals in the fields of allergy, asthma,
and immunology. One of its primary goals is to disseminate cutting-edge
information on asthma and allergy to both physicians and the general public.

Asthma and Allergy Foundation of America (AAFA)
1233 20th Street NW, Suite 402, Washington, DC 20036
1-800-7ASTHMA
www.aafa.org
Newsletter: *The Asthma and Allergy Advance*
The AAFA is a private, non-profit organization dedicated to finding a cure for
and educating the public about asthma and allergies. AAFA offers community
workshops and newsletters for adults and teens with asthma. Their resource
catalog is full of educational information for educators, parents, and children.

Allergy and Asthma Network Mothers of Asthmatics, Inc. (AANMA)
2751 Prosperity Avenue, Suite 150, Fairfax, VA 22031
1-800-878-4403
www.aanma.org
www.breatherville.org
Magazine: *Allergy and Asthma Today*
Newsletter: *The MA Report*
The AANMA is a non-profit community based organization founded by a
parent of a child with asthma. The organization publishes several practical
booklets on asthma and allergy management. Membership in the network
includes a newsletter, magazine, toll-free helpline, and discounts on products.

American Academy of Pediatrics (AAP)
141 N.W. Point Boulevard, Elk Grove Village, IL 60007
1-847-434-4000
www.aap.org
This site has an extensive list of current literature on all phases of asthma. A
wonderful source of information for the entire family.

American College of Allergy, Asthma and Immunology (ACAAI)

85 West Algonquin Road, Suite 550, Arlington Heights, IL 60005

1-800-842-7777

www.acaai.org

The College represents thousands of specially trained physicians in the field of asthma, allergy, and immunology. Educating the public about the state-of-the-art management of allergy and asthma has been one of the organization's primary objectives since its foundation.

American Lung Association (ALA)

61 Broadway, New York, NY 10006

To contact your local chapter, call 1-800-LUNG-USA

www.lungusa.org

Local ALA chapters sponsor the "Open Airways for Schools" elementary school-based asthma education program. The ALA provides information on asthma camps as well as educational materials, speakers, and resources on asthma for all age groups.

Food Allergy and Anaphylaxis Network (FAAN)

11781 Lee Jackson Highway, Suite 160, Fairfax, VA 22033-3309

1-800-929-4040

www.foodallergy.org

The FAAN is dedicated to raising public awareness of food allergies and anaphylaxis along with promoting education and research. A portion of the FAAN's Web site is designed for kids and teens: http://www.fankids.org/

National Heart, Lung, and Blood Institute (NHLBI)

NHLBI Information Center, National Institutes of Health, PO Box 30105, Bethesda, MD 20824-0105

1-301-251-1222

www.nhlbi.nih.gov/guidelines/asthma/asthgdln.htm

The NHLBI is the primary NIH organization responsible for research on asthma and is the sponsor of the NAEPP (National Asthma Education and Prevention Program) discussed in the text at www.nhlbi.nih.gov/about/naepp. Calculate your BMI (body mass index) at www.nhlbisupport.com/bmi. Get information about the NAEPP (National Asthma Education Program Information Center) at www.nhlbi.nih.gov.

National Jewish Medical and Research Center

1400 Jackson Street, Denver, CO 80206

1-303-388-4461

www.asthma.nationaljewish.org

www.library.nationaljewish.org/pathfinders/

Lung Line allows you to speak to a nurse and request that printed information and pamphlets on asthma and allergy be mailed to you: 1-800-222-LUNG

More Useful Web Information

All Allergy. A portal with many links to a variety of organizations involved in all phases of allergy and asthma. There are subjects suitable for younger children and teenagers.

www.allallergy.net

CDC. The Centers for Disease Control and Prevention has a very informative site on asthma. It includes a map of the United States that allows you to "click" on your state to find out what current asthma research programs are being carried out.

www.cdc.gov/asthma/default/html

The CDC also maintains a Web site with the most up-to-date information on influenza and influenza vaccination.

www.cdc.gov/flu

ChestNet. The American College of Chest Physicians' (ACCP) Web site, ChestNet has educational materials on many aspects of asthma, including on how to use inhalers correctly. The ACCP's educational guide for elementary school students will be interesting to teachers and parents alike, and is presented in both English and Spanish.

www.chestnet.org/education/patient/guides

Clinical studies of asthma lists ongoing investigational studies of asthma and how to participate if you are interested.

www.clinicaltrials.gov/ct/gui/cation/FindCondition?ui=D001249&recruiting=true

Consortium on Asthma Camps is a helpful site for campers and their parents.

www.asthma.camps.org

EPA. The Environmental Protection Agency has a bilingual and user-friendly Web site on asthma with special attention to indoor and outdoor air quality. The EPA site also has a section on "Managing Asthma in the School Environment."

www.epa.gov/asthma.index.html

www.epa.gov/iaq/schools/asthma

Global initiative for Asthma (GINA) was launched in 1993 in collaboration with the National Institutes of Health (NIH) and the World Health Organization (WHO). GINA works with asthma experts worldwide to increase understanding of asthma and to improve the lives of people with asthma. *www.ginasthma.org*

Hospital Web sites include the Mayo Clinic's Foundation for Medical Education and Research, and the National Jewish Medical and Research Center. *www.mayoclinic.com* *www.nationaljewish.org*

Medem. An excellent medical library for physicians, patients, and their families. It provides in-depth coverage for a wide variety of medical conditions. *www.medem.com*

MedlinePlus® offers links to reliable health information on asthma from the U.S. National Library of Medicine. The up-to-date information is organized in categories such as "Latest News," "Disease Management," and "Women," to name a few. *www.nlm.nih.gov/medlineplus/asthma.html* Also, *http://www.nlm.nih.gov/medlineplus/asthmainchildren.html* gives the latest information on asthma in children and young people.

National Association of School Nurses. This site contains teaching information on asthma for school staff. 1-207-833-2117 *www.nasn.org*

NCCAM. The National Center for Complementary and Alternative Medicine is a site under the auspices of the National Institutes of Health (NIH). Because complimentary and alternative medicine are areas of great interest and much confusion, if you are interested in ongoing complimentary and alternative medicine research in asthma, this is a good place to start your learning experience. *www.nccam.nih.gov*

Pharmaceutical company–sponsored Web sites are funded by companies that sell asthma and allergy medicines. Examples are: *www.SchoolAsthmaAllergy.com*—sponsored by Schering-Plough *www.respiratoryinstitute.com*—sponsored by GlaxoSmithKline *www.PregancyandAsthma.com*—sponsored by AstraZeneca *www.everydaykidz.com*—sponsored by AstraZeneca

US Food and Drug Administration is a branch of the US Department of Health and Human Sciences and regulates several products including drugs, medical devices, and biologics. It is a good source of information on asthma treatments.

www.fda.gov

www.fda.gov/cder/mdi/drugs.htm reviews the latest on CFC-free HFA inhalers for asthma.

www.fda.gov/cder/mdi/mdifaqs.htm answers questions about albuterol inhalers.

Table A-1   Intermittent Asthma

Classification in children 0–4 years of age
The NAEPP's expert panel classifies four categories of asthma severity. Step 1 treatment is indicated for mild intermittent asthma.
Symptoms
- Daytime symptoms: ≤ 2 days a week
- Nighttime symptoms: none
- Need for short-acting β_2 bronchodilator for symptoms control: ≤ 2 days/week
- Interference with normal activities and daily routine: none

Exacerbations
- From 0 to 1 per year

Treatment ("Step 1")
- All children with asthma should be prescribed inhaled quick-relief short-acting bronchodilator therapy to be used on an as-needed basis. A short-acting inhaled β_2 agonist is the recommended quick-relief agent.
- No daily medication needed.

Any child with mild intermittent asthma can experience exacerbations of their asthma. The exacerbations may be mild, moderate, or even severe, but they are usually brief, lasting from hours to a few days. Treatment of any exacerbation is mandatory and will require additional medication. A short course of oral corticosteroids may be needed. Between exacerbations, a child who has mild intermittent asthma is asymptomatic. There can be long periods of normal lung function without any symptoms between exacerbations.

Classification in children 5–11 years of age
The NAEPP's expert panel classifies four categories of asthma severity. Step 1 treatment is indicated for mild intermittent asthma.
Symptoms
- Daytime symptoms: ≤ 2 days a week
- Nighttime symptoms: ≤ 2 times a month
- Need for short-acting β_2 bronchodilator for symptoms control: ≤ 2 days/week
- Interference with normal activities and daily routine: none

Lung function tests
- Normal forced expiratory volume (FEV_1) between exacerbations
- Forced expiratory volume (FEV_1) ≥ 80% of predicted
- FEV_1/FVC ratio ≥ 85% of predicted

Exacerbations
- From 0 to 2 per year

Treatment ("Step 1")
- All children with asthma should be prescribed inhaled quick-relief short-acting bronchodilator therapy to be used on an as-needed basis. A short-acting inhaled β_2 agonist is the recommended quick-relief agent.
- No daily medication needed.

Any child with mild intermittent asthma can experience exacerbations of their asthma. The exacerbations may be mild, moderate, or even severe, but they are usually brief, lasting from hours to a few days. Treatment of any exacerbation is mandatory and will require additional medication. A short course of oral coticosteroids may be needed. Between exacerbations, measurement of lung function is normal, and a child who has mild intermittent asthma is asymptomatic. There can be long periods of normal lung function without any symptoms between exacerbations.

Classification in youths 12 years and older (and adults)

The NAEPP's expert panel classifies four categories of asthma severity. Step 1 treatment is indicated for mild intermittent asthma.

Symptoms
- Daytime symptoms: $\leq$ 2 days a week
- Nighttime symptoms: $\leq$ 2 times a month
- Need for short-acting β_2 bronchodilator for symptoms control: $\leq$ 2 days/week
- Interference with normal activities and daily routine: none

Lung function tests
- Normal forced expiratory volume (FEV_1) between exacerbations
- Forced expiratory volume (FEV_1) $\geq$ 80% of predicted
- FEV_1/FVC ratio normal

Exacerbations
- From 0 to 2 per year

Treatment ("Step 1")
- All youths with asthma should be prescribed inhaled quick-relief short-acting bronchodilator therapy to be used on an as-needed basis. A short-acting inhaled β_2 agonist is the recommended quick-relief agent.
- No daily medication needed.

Any youth with mild intermittent asthma can experience exacerbations of their asthma. The exacerbations may be mild, moderate, or even severe, but they are usually brief, lasting from hours to a few days. Treatment of any exacerbation is mandatory and will require additional medication. A short course of oral corticosteroids may be needed. Between exacerbations, measurement lung function is normal, and the youth who has mild intermittent asthma is asymptomatic. There can be long periods of normal lung function without any symptoms between exacerbations.

Table A-2   Mild Persistent Asthma

Classification in children 0–4 years of age

The NAEPP's expert panel classifies four categories of asthma severity. Step 2 treatment is indicated for mild persistent asthma.

Symptoms
- Daytime symptoms: > 2 days a week, but not daily
- Nighttime symptoms: > 1 to 2 times a month
- Need for short-acting β_2 bronchodilator for symptoms control: > 2 days a week, but not daily
- Interference with normal activities and daily routine: minor limitation

Exacerbations
- 2 or more in 6 months requiring oral steroids, or 4 or more wheezing episodes per year

Treatment ("Step 2")
- All children with asthma should be prescribed inhaled quick-relief bronchodilator therapy to be used on an as-needed basis. A short-acting inhaled β_2 agonist is the recommended quick-relief agent.
- Daily medication is required. In most cases, low-dose inhaled anti-inflammatory medication is preferred. Montelukast or cromolyn can be alternatives.
- Consultation with an asthma specialist may be considered.

Any child with mild persistent asthma can experience exacerbations of asthma. The exacerbations may be mild, moderate, or even severe. Treatment of any exacerbation is mandatory and will require additional medication. A course of oral corticosteroids may be needed.

Classification in children 5–11 years of age

The NAEPP's expert panel classifies four categories of asthma severity. Step 2 treatment is indicated for mild persistent asthma.

Symptoms
- Daytime symptoms: > 2 days a week, but not daily
- Nighttime symptoms: > 3–4 times a month
- Need for short-acting β_2 bronchodilator for symptoms control: > 2 days a week, but not daily
- Interference with normal activities and daily routine: minor limitation

Lung function tests
- Forced expiratory volume (FEV_1) ≥ 80% of predicted
- FEV_1/FVC ratio greater than 80% of predicted

Exacerbations
- More than 2 per year

Treatment ("Step 2")
- All children with asthma should be prescribed inhaled quick-relief bronchodilator therapy to be used on an as-needed basis. A short-acting inhaled β_2 agonist is the recommended quick-relief agent.
- Daily medication is required. In most cases, low-dose inhaled anti-inflammatory medication is preferred. Pills such as leukotriene modifiers or sustained-release theophylline tablets can be alternatives along with cromolyn and nedocromil.

Any child with mild persistent asthma can experience exacerbations of asthma. The exacerbations may be mild, moderate, or even severe. Treatment of any exacerbation is mandatory and will require additional medication. A course of oral corticosteroids may be needed.

Classification in youths 12 years and older (and adults)

The NAEPP's expert panel classifies four categories of asthma severity. Step 2 treatment is indicated for mild intermittent asthma.

Symptoms
- Daytime symptoms: > 2 days a week, but not daily
- Nighttime symptoms: > 3–4 times a month
- Need for short-acting β_2 bronchodilator for symptoms control: > 2 days a week, but not daily
- Interference with normal activities and daily routine: minor limitation

Lung function tests
- Forced expiratory volume (FEV_1) ≥ 80% of predicted
- FEV_1/FVC ratio ≥ 80% of predicted

Exacerbations
- More than 2 per year

Treatment ("Step 2")
- Daily medication is required. In most cases, low-dose inhaled anti-inflammatory medication is preferred. Pills such as leukotriene modifiers or sustained-release theophylline tablets can be alternatives along with cromolyn and nedocromil.
- No daily medication needed.

Any youth with mild persistent asthma can experience exacerbations of asthma. The exacerbations may be mild, moderate, or even severe. Treatment of any exacerbation is mandatory and will require additional medication. A course of oral coticosteroids may be needed.

Table A-3   Moderate Persistent Asthma

Classification in children 0–4 years of age
The NAEPP's expert panel classifies four categories of asthma severity. Step 3 treatment is indicated for moderate persistent asthma.
Symptoms
- Daytime symptoms: daily
- Nighttime symptoms: > 3–4 times a month
- Need for short-acting β_2 bronchodilator for symptoms control: daily
- Interference with normal activities and daily routine: some limitation

Exacerbations
- Two or more in 6 months requiring oral steroids, or 4 or more wheezing episodes per year

Treatment ("Step 3")
- All children with asthma should be prescribed inhaled quick-relief bronchodilator therapy to be used on an as-needed basis in addition to daily control medicine. A short-acting inhaled β_2 agonist is the recommended quick-relief agent.
- Daily medication is required. The treating physician will prescribe a regimen based on the patient's individual asthma characteristics. Medium-dose inhaled corticosteroid anti-inflammatory medication is preferred.
- Consultation with an asthma specialist is recommended.

Any child with mild persistent asthma can experience exacerbations of asthma. The exacerbations may be mild, moderate, or even severe. Treatment of any exacerbation is mandatory and will require additional medication. A course of oral corticosteroids may be needed.

Classification in children 5–11 years of age
The NAEPP's expert panel classifies four categories of asthma severity. Step 3 treatment is indicated for moderate persistent asthma.
Symptoms
- Daytime symptoms: daily
- Nighttime symptoms: > 1 night a week, but not nightly
- Need for short-acting β_2 bronchodilator for symptoms control: daily
- Interference with normal activities and daily routine: some limitation

Lung function tests
- Forced expiratory volume (FEV_1) = 60% to 80% predicted
- FEV_1/FVC ratio = 75%–80%

Exacerbations
- More than 2 per year

Treatment ("Step 3")
- All children with asthma should be prescribed inhaled quick-relief bronchodilator therapy to be used on an as-needed basis in addition to daily control medicine. A short-acting inhaled β_2 agonist is the recommended quick-relief agent.
- Daily medication is required. The treating physician will prescribe a regimen based on the patient's individual asthma characteristics. One recommended regimen includes a medium-dose inhaled corticosteroid along with a long-acting β_2 agonist.
- Refer children with moderate persistent asthma to a physician who is an asthma specialist.

Anyone with moderate persistent asthma can experience exacerbations of their asthma. The exacerbations tend to last for several days. Treatment of any exacerbation is mandatory and will require additional medication, such as oral corticosteroids.

Classification in youths 12 years and older (and adults)
The NAEPP's expert panel classifies four categories of asthma severity. Step 3 treatment is indicated for moderate persistent asthma.

Symptoms
  • Daytime symptoms: daily
  • Nighttime symptoms: > 1 night a week, but not nightly
  • Need for short-acting β_2 bronchodilator for symptoms control: daily
  • Interference with normal activities and daily routine: some limitation

Lung function tests
  • Forced expiratory volume (FEV_1) = greater than 60% and less than 80% predicted
  • FEV_1/FVC ratio = reduced by 5% from normal

Exacerbations
  • More than 2 per year

Treatment ("Step 3")
  • All youths with asthma should be prescribed inhaled quick-relief bronchodilator therapy to be used on an as-needed basis in addition to daily control medicine. A short-acting inhaled β_2 agonist is the recommended quick-relief agent.
  • Daily medication is required. The treating physician will prescribe a regimen based on the patient's individual asthma characteristics. One recommended regimen includes a medium-dose inhaled corticosteroid or a low-dose inhaled corticosteroid combined with a long-acting inhaled β_2 agonist bronchodilator. Alternatives can be reviewed with the treating physician and include a low-dose inhaled corticosteroid combined with a second oral medicine.
  • Consider referral of youths with moderate persistent asthma to a physician who is an asthma specialist.

Anyone with moderate persistent asthma can experience exacerbations of their asthma. The exacerbations tend to last for several days. Treatment of any exacerbation is mandatory and will require additional medication such as oral corticosteroids.

Table A-4   Severe Persistent Asthma

Classification in children 0–4 years of age
The NAEPP's expert panel classifies four categories of asthma severity.
Step 4–6 treatment is indicated for severe persistent asthma.
Symptoms
- Daytime symptoms: daily, throughout the day
- Nighttime symptoms: > more than once a week
- Need for short-acting β_2 bronchodilator for symptoms control: several times daily
- Interference with normal activities and daily routine: very limited

Exacerbations
- Two or more in 6 months requiring oral steroids, or 4 or more wheezing episodes per year

Treatment ("Step 4, Step 5, or Step 6")
- All children with asthma should be prescribed inhaled quick-relief bronchodilator therapy to be used on an as-needed basis addition to daily control medicine. A short-acting inhaled β_2 agonist is the recommended quick-relief agent.
- Daily medication is required. The treating physician will prescribe a regimen based on the patient's individual asthma characteristics. One recommended regimen includes a high-dose inhaled corticosteroid possibly combined with either montelukast or a long-acting inhaled β_2 agonist bronchodilator.
- Youths with moderate persistent asthma should be under the care of an asthma specialist.
- Consultation with an asthma specialist is recommended.

Anyone with moderate persistent asthma can experience exacerbations of their asthma. The exacerbations tend to last for several days. Treatment of any exacerbation is mandatory and will require additional medication such as oral corticosteroids.

Classification in children 5–11 years of age

The NAEPP's expert panel classifies four categories of asthma severity. Step 4–6 treatment is indicated for severe persistent asthma.

Symptoms
- Daytime symptoms: daily, throughout the day
- Nighttime symptoms: often nightly, 7 times a week
- Need for short-acting β_2 bronchodilator for symptoms control: several times daily
- Interference with normal activities and daily routine: very limited

Lung function tests
- Forced expiratory volume (FEV_1) < 60% of predicted
- FEV_1/FVC ratio < 75% of predicted

Exacerbations
- More than 2 per year

Treatment ("Step 4, Step 5, or Step 6")
- All children with asthma should be prescribed inhaled quick-relief bronchodilator therapy to be used on an as-needed basis in addition to daily control medicine. A short-acting inhaled β_2 agonist is the recommended quick-relief agent.
- Daily medication is required. The treating physician will prescribe a regimen based on the patient's individual asthma characteristics. One suggested regimen includes a high-dose inhaled corticosteroid combined with a long-acting inhaled β_2 agonist bronchodilator. Some youths will also need a daily dose of oral corticosteroid. Alternatives can be discussed with the physician. The treating physician may also suggest the addition of Omalizumab (in older children) if allergy is playing a significant role in asthma.
- Children with moderate persistent asthma should be under the care of an asthma specialist.

Anyone with moderate persistent asthma can experience exacerbations of their asthma. The exacerbations tend to last for several days. Treatment of any exacerbation is mandatory and will require additional medication such as oral corticosteroids.

Classification in youths 12 years and older (and adults)
The NAEPP's expert panel classifies four categories of asthma severity. Step 4–6 treatment is indicated for severe persistent asthma.
Symptoms
  • Daytime symptoms, throughout the day
  • Nighttime symptoms: often nightly, 7 times a week
  • Need for short-acting β_2 bronchodilator for symptoms control: several times daily
  • Interference with normal activities and daily routine: very limited
Lung function tests
  • Forced expiratory volume (FEV_1) < 60% of predicted
  • FEV_1/FVC ratio = reduced by more than 5% from normal
Exacerbations
  • More than 2 per year
Treatment ("Step 4, Step 5, or Step 6")
  • All youths with asthma should be prescribed inhaled quick-relief bronchodilator therapy to be used on an as-needed basis in addition to daily control medicine. A short-acting inhaled β_2 agonist is the recommended quick-relief agent.
  • Daily medication is required. The treating physician will prescribe a regimen based on the patient's individual asthma characteristics. One suggested regimen includes a high-dose inhaled corticosteroid combined with a long-acting inhaled β_2 agonist bronchodilator. Some youths will also need a daily dose of oral corticosteroid. Alternatives can be discussed with the physician. The treating physician may also suggest the addition of Omalizumab if allergy is playing a significant role in asthma.
  • Youths with moderate persistent asthma should be under the care of an asthma specialist.

Anyone with moderate persistent asthma can experience exacerbations of their asthma. The exacerbations tend to last for several days. Treatment of any exacerbation is mandatory and will require additional medication such as oral corticosteroids.

Glossary

A

Actuation: The action that releases a dose of medication from a metered-dose inhaler (MDI).

Acute: Short-lived, brief, sudden, not drawn out. *Chronic* is the opposite of acute. A virus such as influenza will cause an acute illness that may last a few weeks. Asthma is an example of a non-acute or chronic condition. Although its symptoms may recede, asthma lasts indefinitely.

Agonist: A drug that exerts its actions by combining with specific sites (called receptors) in the body. Albuterol, for example, attaches to the lungs' β_2 receptors. By attaching to the β_2 receptors, albuterol exerts its bronchodilatory effects and causes narrowed bronchial passages to dilate, or open up. Stimulation of the lung β_2 receptors leads to rapid relief of wheezing, tightness, and bronchoconstriction. Medicines such as albuterol are called β (beta) agonists since they fit the β_2 receptor and exert their effects through activation of the receptor sites.

Air trapping: A potentially reversible phenomenon that develops in the lungs of patients with poorly controlled or uncontrolled asthma. Air trapping can be detected on chest CT scans but is best assessed by pulmonary function test measurements. Air trapping reflects uneven lung emptying as certain areas of lung take longer to empty of air before they fill up again with the next breath. Any process that effectively narrows the caliber of the bronchial passageways can lead to air trapping. Examples of those processes include bronchoconstriction as well as accumulation of mucus in the bronchial tubes.

Albuterol: A β_2 agonist medication that acts on the respiratory passages to cause bronchodilatation. It is classified as a quick-relief, fast-acting medicine and is extensively prescribed in the treatment of bronchial asthma. Albuterol should be taken to relieve earliest symptoms of chest discomfort, cough, wheeze, or sensations of tightness due to asthma. It is usually delivered either by a nebulizer or by a metered dose inhaler, but an oral form also exists.

Allergen: An agent that is able to produce an abnormal (allergic) response in a susceptible individual when that person becomes exposed to the agent. An allergen is usually a protein and can be of various origins. Foods, pollen, and animal dander, for example, can act as allergens in susceptible individuals, as can substances of plant or animal origin. Specific examples of common allergens include peanut, penicillin, ragweed, and cat dander. Allergens are not universal; they lead to an allergic response only in susceptible persons. Allergens may be asthma triggers for certain children who have both asthma and allergy.

Allergenic: Capable of causing an abnormal (allergic) response in a susceptible (allergic) individual. Some substances are considered to be more allergenic than others, meaning that those substances are known to more frequently lead to allergy symptoms in general. Pediatricians, for example, know which foods are more inherently allergenic than others, so they generally advise introducing them later in a child's diet, and only very gradually at first. Tree nuts, fish, and eggs are more allergenic in very young children than other foods such as rice, banana, beef, or green beans, so they are added to the menu only as children grow older.

Allergic rhinitis: A manifestation of allergy expressed as nasal symptoms with itching, runny nose, and congestion. When caused by seasonal airborne allergens, allergic rhinitis is sometimes referred to as hay fever or rose fever. *See* Rhinitis.

Allergist: A physician specialized in the diagnosis and treatment of persons with allergies. Many practicing allergists in the United States have special training first in pediatrics, followed by additional qualifications in allergy. Although they treat patients in all age groups, pediatric allergists have a particular interest and expertise in allergies in children. Because many (if not most) allergies are first di-

agnosed in childhood, it makes sense to have the dual medical background.

Allergy: The body's physical reaction to certain external substances known as allergens. Allergens are harmless to nonallergic persons. Allergy involves the body's production of a specific antibody in direct response to a specific allergen. The result of the allergy–antibody interaction includes inflammatory and immune changes. Those changes, in turn, lead to symptoms that may affect the eyes (allergic conjunctivitis), nose (allergic rhinitis), sinuses (allergic sinusitis), skin (eczema, hives, atopic dermatitis), and lungs (allergic asthma).

Allergy testing: Allergy tests can be obtained by two general methods: either "directly" on the patient or "indirectly" through a blood sample (RAST®) drawn from a vein. Direct tests include two different techniques: the prick (or prick-puncture) test and the intradermal test. Direct tests are the most sensitive way of determining whether a person has become sensitized to a specific allergen (such as peanut, cat, or ragweed). Direct tests are performed most often on either the forearm (for prick-puncture testing) or the upper arm (for intradermal testing).

Alveolar-capillary membrane: The alveolar-capillary membrane is the interface between the alveolar wall and the blood circulation. It permits rapid, nearly instantaneous exchange of oxygen, carbon dioxide, and other gases between the air-filled alveoli and the body's blood circulation running through the capillary blood vessels. The alveolar-capillary membrane becomes damaged in diseases such as emphysema, but is unaffected by well-controlled asthma.

Alveolus (pl. alveoli): An alveolus is a lung's air sac. Oxygen is exchanged for carbon dioxide in the lung alveoli. A dense network of capillary vessels surrounds each alveolus. The close arrangement allows for very rapid exchange (or diffusion) of oxygen from alveolus to capillary, and of carbon dioxide from capillary to alveolus. A healthy adult human lung contains approximately 300 million alveoli. The average diameter of a human alveolus is one quarter of a millimeter. The total alveolar surface available for gas exchange in a healthy adult approximates 100 meters^2, which is about the size of a tennis court.

Anabolic steroids: Compounds normally produced by the body in health that have the capacity to increase muscle mass, among other effects. Athletes have sometimes inappropriately taken anabolic steroids as supplements in order to build strength, endurance, and muscle mass. Anabolic steroids are unrelated to the corticosteroids used in asthma treatment but are sometimes confused with such medications because of the common use of "steroids" to refer to both types of compounds.

Anaphylaxis: The most severe form of an allergic reaction or response. If untreated, anaphylaxis can be fatal. The term *anaphylactic shock* is sometimes used to describe the most dramatic and serious form of anaphylaxis. Anaphylaxis usually involves several organ systems, including the cardiovascular system, skin, respiratory system, and gastrointestinal tract. Symptoms include a dangerous drop in blood pressure (hypotension), hives (urticaria) with itching and rash, respiratory distress and wheezing, throat tightness, nausea, vomiting, and abdominal pain. Immediate emergency treatment is imperative. Persons at risk for the development of anaphylaxis, such as persons known to have had a prior significant allergic reaction to peanut or bee stings, should always have injectable epinephrine on hand. If an anaphylactic reaction were to occur, prompt injection of epinephrine under the skin is literally lifesaving.

Antagonist: Something that opposes or resists the action of another. In medicine, an antagonist is a compound that prevents the effects or actions of a different compound, e.g., antihistamine antagonizes the effects of histamine.

Antibody: A protein molecule produced in blood or tissues in direct response to a foreign substance or antigen. A specific antigen leads to the production of a corresponding specific antibody. The production of antibody can be beneficial or deleterious, depending on the circumstances. Antibody made in response to an infectious agent, such as measles, will protect against a second measles infection or a recurrence. Antibody made in response to common environmental agents, such as pollens, grasses, mold, and animal dander, may lead to the development of allergy. Only susceptible persons (allergic or atopic individuals) will actually produce antibody against common allergens. The presence of antibody in response to a particular antigen is referred to as *sensitization* to that particular antigen. When such a person goes on to develop an allergy to that allergen, the antibody is usually of the immunoglobulin E (IgE) class.

Antihistamine: The class of medicines that counteract the effects of histamine by blocking histamine receptors on cells, which in turn prevents symptoms such as sneeze, runny nose, or watering eyes. Antihistimines are most effective when taken before symptoms develop.

Aspirin: Originally Bayer's trademark for acetylsalicylic acid, a medicine with anti-inflammatory properties. Rather than refer uniquely to the Bayer brand, aspirin now designates any preparation of acetylsalicylic acid. Aspirin has analgesic and antipyretic properties; it is prescribed to relieve pain and fever. Because of its anti-inflammatory actions, it is also used to treat rheumatoid arthritis, juvenile rheumatoid arthritis, and many forms of heart disease. Its use is contraindicated in any person with aspirin-sensitive asthma in whom it may trigger wheezing and bronchospasm (exacerbation).

Asthma: Originally derived from the phrase "difficult breathing." Asthma is a chronic respiratory condition characterized by breathing symptoms of varying intensity and frequency. Asthma has a strong genetic (inherited) basis, although environmental influences also play an important role. Asthma frequently goes hand-in-hand with allergy, especially in younger age groups.

Asthmagenic: A situation or substance that has the potential to trigger or bring on asthma symptoms, e.g., exercise, exposure to cold air, or response to an allergen.

Asymptomatic: Without any manifestations or symptoms of disease or illness. The major goal of asthma treatment is to achieve an asymptomatic state so that the person with asthma experiences no symptoms and is able to lead a full and productive life.

Atopy/Atopic: Atopy is an inherited predisposition to the development of allergic conditions such as hay fever, eczema, allergic rhinitis, and even certain forms of asthma. A person with evidence of atopy is said to be atopic.

Auscultation: The process of listening to the sounds of air moving in and out of the breathing passages. Auscultation is performed by the examiner placing a stethoscope on the skin overlying the lungs and having the patient breathe in and out.

B

Barrel-chest deformity: Development of a deformed chest that can occur as a result of inadequate treatment of severe chronic asthma. Chronic air trapping eventually causes the bones of the thorax to assume a rounded, barrel-like shape.

Baseline hyperreactivity: Baseline hyperreactivity (BHR) is a key characteristic of asthma. BHR refers to asthmatic lungs' innate tendency to react to certain stimuli with an inflammatory response that in turn leads to typical asthma symptoms, including breathlessness, chest tightness, breathing discomfort, cough, and wheezing. Asthma and a state of increased baseline hyperreactivity go hand-in-hand. BHR can be conceptualized as the asthmatic lungs' greater sensitivity to inhaled substances that would produce no such effect in a healthy person who does not have asthma. Persons with asthma, for example, might start to experience uncomfortable breathing when entering a room where people are smoking cigarettes or when running outdoors to catch a bus in subzero temperatures. Their friends, who are accompanying them to the party or sprinting alongside to catch the bus, experience no respiratory discomfort in the same situations. Physicians can assess BHR using a special pulmonary function test called the methacholine challenge (or bronchoprovocation) test. Scientists and physicians hope that future research into BHR might yield treatments that would modify or lessen the increased BHR that is characteristic of asthma.

Body mass index (BMI): A mathematical formula based on height and weight. BMI is a tool used in population studies of obesity because of its ease of measurement. The BMI in most individuals correlates to measures of body fat. To calculate your BMI, you can use either metric or conventional American units. You need to know your weight measured in kilograms or pounds, and your height measured in meters or inches. Then use one of the formulae below:

**BMI = weight in kilograms ÷ (height in meters × height in meters)

**BMI = (weight in pounds ÷ height in inches ÷ height in inches) × 703.

Obesity can be defined based on a person's BMI. An adult with a BMI of between 25 and 30 is considered overweight, and an adult with a BMI of 30 or greater meets criteria for a diagnosis of obesity. Note that BMI is used differently in children and adolescents. The interpretation of BMI values in children and adolescents requires an adjustment for age.

Bronchial passageways: The breathing tubes of the lungs.

Bronchiole: The fine, tapered, thin-walled breathing passages that branch and extend from the bronchi and end in the alveolar air sacs.

Bronchiolitis: An inflammation of the tiniest bronchial tubes. Bronchiolitis can be secondary to an infection (infectious bronchiolitis) or caused by a noninfectious cause such as cigarette smoking (smoker's bronchiolitis).

Bronchitis: An inflammation of the lining of the larger bronchial tubes. Bronchitis can be acute, such as from infection, or chronic, such as in the case of tobacco abuse. Chronic obstructive bronchitis is the correct American term for the cigarette-related type of chronic obstructive pulmonary disease that demonstrates obstructive dysfunction on pulmonary function tests, and that causes symptoms of cough, mucus production, breathlessness, and episodes of wheezing.

Bronchoconstriction: An abnormal narrowing of the air passages. Bronchoconstriction is a prominent characteristic of asthma and is caused by an increased inflammatory response in the lung.

Bronchodilator: An agent that leads to widening, or opening up, of the lung air passages; the reverse of broncho-constriction. Bronchodilator medicines improve breathing and relieve asthma symptoms by opening and restoring the caliber of abnormally narrowed (constricted) bronchi.

Bronchoprovocation test: A specialized pulmonary function test that asseses for the presence of baseline hyperreactivity and that can be helpful in the diagnostic evaluation of suspected asthma. Both methacholine challenge testing and cold-air exercise challenge are examples of bronchoprovocation tests.

Bronchospasm: Abnormal contraction of the bronchial smooth muscles. *See* bronchoconstriction.

Bronchus (pl. bronchi): A lung breathing passage or tube. The trachea splits at the level of the carina into the right and left mainstem bronchi. The right mainstem bronchus leads air to and from the entire right lung. The left mainstem bronchus leads air to and from the entire left lung. The mainstem bronchi further subdivide into bronchial tubes that lead to the subdivisions of each lung. The bronchial tubes eventually branch out into smaller and narrower air passages called bronchioles before ending in alveoli.

C

Caffeine: A compound found naturally in coffee and tea, and added to other beverages such as soda or energy drinks.

It is also added some medications, such as those used for treatment of pain or headache. Caffeine has several effects in the body. It is a weak lung bronchodilator and a central nervous system stimulant, and increases mental alertness and wakefulness. Caffeine acts as a mild kidney diuretic, leading to an increase in urine excretion.

Capillary: A capillary is a tiny, thin-walled blood vessel. The word is derived from *capillus*, the Latin word for hair. The lungs' capillaries play a crucial role in health as part of the alveolar–capillary membrane, absorbing oxygen into the body and getting rid of carbon dioxide.

Carbon dioxide: Carbon dioxide (CO_2) is an odorless, colorless gas produced as a waste by-product of the body's metabolism. Carbon dioxide is normally excreted by the lungs and should not be confused with carbon monoxide (symbol: CO), which is a poisonous, odorless gas that, when inhaled, can lead to carbon monoxide poisoning.

Carina: The split where the lungs' trachea divides into two branches: the right mainstem bronchus and the left mainstem bronchus. Each bronchus leads air to the right and left lung respectively.

Chlorofluorocarbons (CFCs): Chemical propellants previously used in the manufacture of metered-dose inhalers. The manufacture and use of CFCs are now banned. A time-limited exception (due to expire in 2008) has been granted for certain inhalers until an equivalent replacement formulation is in production and available to patients.

Chromosome: Cellular microscopic structures that contain groupings of DNA. Chromosomes carry genetic information, or genes, in their DNA. All human cells (except a female's mature ova and a male's sperm cells) contain in their center, or nucleus, a total of 46 chromosomes, divided in 23 pairs. An individual's 46 chromosomes constitute their genome. Half of the chromosomes are inherited from the father (through the sperm cell's 23 chromosomes) and half from the mother (through the mature ova's 23 chromosomes).

Chronic: Longstanding, lingering, or expected to last indefinitely; opposite of acute. Asthma and hypertension are considered chronic illnesses, for example. Although both respond very well to treatment and can be readily brought under control, they still last indefinitely from a medical perspective.

Chronic obstructive bronchitis: Chronic obstructive bronchitis is the technically correct medical term for the cigarette-related type of chronic obstructive pulmonary disease that demonstrates obstructive dysfunction on pulmonary function tests and causes symptoms of cough, mucus production, breathlessness, and episodes of wheezing.

Chronic obstructive pulmonary disease: A lung disease of adults which targets the airways. In COPD, the airways and air sacs lose their shape and affect the flow of air.

Compliance: The consistent daily use of medications or treatments in accordance with a doctor's instructions or prescription. Also called adherence.

Constriction: Narrowing; the opposite of dilatation. *See also* bronchoconstriction.

Corticosteroids: Hormones that are normally produced in very small quantities by the body's adrenal glands. Corticosteroids play a role in regulating blood pressure and in maintaining the body's salt and water balance. Corticosteroids have been synthesized in the laboratory. They are useful medicines when prescribed in the treatment of inflammatory conditions. Corticosteroids in inhaled form are a key medication used to treat asthma in all age groups.

CT scan: Computerized tomography is a 3-dimensional imaging technique that provides very precise anatomic detail using x-ray technology. Images of the sinuses and lungs produced by CT scanning provide physicians with accurate information about how those structures look.

Cyanosis: An abnormal physical examination finding that correlates with abnormally low levels of blood oxygen. Cyanosis is a bluish discoloration best detected in the nail beds (under the fingernails) and around the lips.

Cystic fibrosis: A congenital metabolic disorder that primarily involves the lungs and the gastrointestinal system. Children with cystic fibrosis produce thick mucus that causes obstruction in the pancreas, liver, intestines, and lungs. Early diagnosis and treatment are critical factors for insuring the long-term survival of children with this condition.

D

Densensitization: Reduction or elimination of an allergic sensitivity or reaction to a specific allergen. Immunotherapy ("allergy shots") is generally used to achieve densensitization in patients with allergies.

Differential diagnosis: The process of considering different conditions or diseases that could be responsible for a patient's symptoms. After reviewing the patient's history, findings of the physical examination, and laboratory and test data, a physician will generate a list of differential diagnoses. Each diagnosis on the list is a "possible" and some are more likely than others.

Diffusion: The process in which gases and liquids intermingle until a state of balance or equilibrium is obtained. During respiration, inhaled oxygen gas diffuses from the alveolus into capillary blood (a liquid) in the lung, while carbon dioxide gas diffuses out of the capillary blood into the alveolus. Diffusion of oxygen and of carbon dioxide occurs extremely rapidly across the alveolar-capillary membrane in healthy lungs. Several disease states can interfere with the diffusing capacity of the lung. Emphysema, for example, destroys normal lung. As diffusion becomes more and more impaired, emphysematous lungs can no longer supply enough oxygen for the body's needs. Supplemental (extra) oxygen is sometimes required in the treatment of advanced emphysema, and is administered continuously through tubing and nasal prongs. Pulmonary function testing (PFT) includes an assessment of the lung's diffusion capacity in a test called, appropriately, *diffusion*. Although diffusion can be impaired during a significant exacerbation of asthma, diffusion measured on PFTs is generally within normal or predicted values in asthma.

Dilatation: An opening or widening; the opposite of constriction. *See also* bronchoconstriction.

Dry powder inhaler (DPI): A DPI is a newer method of delivering medication directly to the lungs and respiratory passages. DPIs are supplanting traditional MDIs because of their ease of use, convenience, and good patient acceptance. Most children can learn to use DPIs effectively beginning at age 6. Several different classes of respiratory medicines are available in DPI form, including inhaled corticosteroids, long-acting β_2 agonists, and anticholinergic bronchodilators.

Dust mites: Dust mites are common household antigens. They are microscopic living organisms found indoors in tempered climates, especially in mattresses, bedding, and upholstered furniture. Dust mites live off scales of human skin. A common cause of allergy and asthma exacerbation, their numbers can be greatly reduced or nearly eliminated by straightforward control measures in the home. Some of those measures include adjustment of the home's humidity level, encasement of all bedding in special covers, laundering bedding in hot water on a regular basis, and eliminating stuffed animals along with certain types of furniture, floor coverings, and draperies.

Dyspnea: An abnormal awareness of breathing; a kind of breathlessness. The act of breathing should be automatic and comfortable. Dyspnea is a classic symptom of asthma and should lessen once treatment is prescribed.

E

Eczema: Eczema is an allergic skin condition and is also known as *atopic dermatitis*. In babies, eczema often involves the cheeks and the diaper area, whereas in older children a distribution behind the elbow creases and the area behind the knees is classic. Eczema can be very itchy and drying.

Effector cells: Specialized white blood cells (such as macrophages, T cells, B cells, and activated mast cells) that interact and release mediators that create the typical symptoms of an allergic response.

Emphysema: One of the chronic obstructive pulmonary diseases that affects adults. Cigarette smoking is a significant risk factor for the development of emphysema.

Endogenous steroids: Steroids normally produced in health by the body's adrenal glands. *See* corticosteroids.

Endoscopic examination: An examination using an endoscope, which is a tool used for examining a hollow organ or canal such as the esophagus or stomach. The endoscope transmits light into the organ and provides the physician with an image of the interior or the organ.

Environmental control: One of the three components of a comprehensive management and treatment program for children with asthma. Specifically, the term refers to the avoidance or elimination from the home, school, or work environment of those substances, allergens, or irritants that are responsible for a patient's symptoms. Common targets of environmental control include dust mites, household pets, and the use of wood-burning fireplaces.

Eosinophils: White blood cells involved in combating infection by parasites as well as playing a role in allergy and asthma.

Epidemiologic: Based on the study of populations or large groups of people.

Epinephrine: A naturally occurring hormone produced by the human adrenal glands. A synthetic form (adrenaline) is used to treat severe allergic reactions (anaphylaxis) and life-threatening asthma.

Estrogens: A group of female hormones synthesized chiefly by the ovaries. Estrogens stimulate the development and maintenance of the female secondary sexual characteristics.

Exacerbation: A flare of disease activity or disease symptoms. An exacerbation of asthma can be caused by a viral infection, for example, and leads to increased symptoms of cough, mucus, chest tightness, and wheezing.

Expiration: The action of breathing air out of the lungs, called exhaling. The respiratory cycle has two parts: inspiration and expiration.

Expiratory: Refers to breathing out.

F

FEV₁: Forced expiratory volume in one second, which is a subtest of the spirometry portion of the pulmonary function tests. Both the FEV_1 and a second measurement, the FEV_1/FVC ratio, are used to diagnose asthma and to assess and follow response to treatment.

Fulminant: Occurring suddenly, with great intensity and severity.

G

Gas exchange: Refers to the process by which oxygen and carbon dioxide enter and leave the body through the lungs' alveolar capillary membrane.

Gastroenterologist: A physician who is a specialist in diseases involving the gastrointestinal tract. Commonly referred to as a "GI specialist".

Gastroesophageal reflux disease (GERD): A medical condition that often leads to heartburn, and may also significantly worsen underlying asthma. GERD, or more simply *reflux*, is usually treated with a combination of dietary changes and medicine.

Gene: A unit of heredity made up of a sequence of DNA. Genes are the basic unit of inheritance. Each gene occupies a specific place (locus) on a chromosome. They are capable of duplicating themselves each time a cell divides, and genes determine a particular characteristic or trait.

Genetic: Related to a gene or a gene product. A genetic trait is an inherited characteristic that is passed from parent to child at conception.

Global Initiative for Asthma (GINA): A program launched in 1993 in collaboration with the National Heart, Lung, and Blood Institute, National Institutes of Health, USA, and the World Health Organization. GINA's program is determined and its guidelines for asthma care are shaped by committees made up of leading asthma experts from around the world.

Glucose intolerance: A condition in which the body shows some degree of resistance to insulin, so it can't move glucose into cells efficiently and utilize it as an efficient body fuel. This condition can range from "prediabetes," in which high blood glucose is notably above normal after a fast but below levels diagnostic of diabetes, to Type 2 diabetes.

H

High Efficiency Particulate Air (HEPA) filter: An air filter that meets very stringent filtration requirements. HEPA filters are capable of trapping particles of very small size, including common indoor allergens and even certain microorganisms that pose a risk to human health. HEPA filters are used in industrial settings and in hospitals. In hospitals, for example, HEPA filters are incorporated into the ventilation and exhaust systems of operating suites and isolation rooms. HEPA filters are occasionally recommended in the home as part of environmental control measures in treatment of allergy.

Histamine: A naturally occurring chemical that exerts effects on muscle, blood capillaries, and stomach secretions by attaching to H_1 and H_2 receptors in the body. Most of the body's histamine is located in mast cells, which are a type of white blood cell. When histamine is released from mast cells as occurs during an allergic reaction, the released histamine attaches to the histamine receptor and that combination causes an inflammatory response that can include bronchoconstriction in the lung (from constriction of the muscles that encircle the bronchial tubes) and wheezing, runny nose, tearing, hives, itching, and increased stomach acid production. Medicines of the antihistamine class block the attachment of histamine to the histamine receptors and effectively neutralize the inflammatory response mediated by histamine.

Hormone: A chemical substance produced in the body by specialized organs called endocrine glands. Once synthesized, hormones circulate in the bloodstream and regulate different body functions. Insulin is a hormone, for example. It is produced in the pancreas gland and enters the blood circulation where it exerts profound effects on glucose (sugar) and carbohydrate metabolism.

Hydrofluoroalkane (HFA): Medically inert substances that are used as propellants in metered-dose inhalers and meet chlorofluorocarbon-free criteria.

Hygiene hypothesis: A theory that links exposure to "dirty" environments and to certain infectious agents at specific times in early childhood to a decreased risk for the development of asthma. The hypothesis attempts to connect the increasing prevalence of childhood asthma with the concurrent decreased prevalence of infections in childhood.

Hyperinflation: Lung overdistention; sometimes used interchangeably with air trapping, as air trapping results in hyperinflation. Uncontrolled or poorly controlled asthma may lead to hyperinflation, which should abate and reverse with treatment.

Hyperreactivity: With respect to asthma, refers to asthmatic lungs' greater sensitivity to inhaled substances that would produce no effect in a healthy person without asthma.

Hyposensitization: A term used to indicate one possible (favorable) outcome of allergen immunotherapy ("allergy shots"). It refers to a decrease, but not total elimination, of a person's ability to develop allergic symptoms to a specific allergen, which occurs as a result of an immunotherapy regimen.

Hypoxia: Refers to decreased and abnormally low levels of oxygen in the bloodstream.

I

Immune system: The primary defense system of the body, the immune system is responsible for providing protection against bacteria, viruses, cancer, and any proteins that are foreign to the body. The system is composed of the thymus gland, the bone marrow, the lymph nodes (glands), the spleen, and specialized lymphoid tissue located in the intestinal tract. Without a properly functioning immune system, we would not be able to survive.

Immunoglobulin E (IgE): IgE is a type of immunoglobulin that increases and is produced in greater quantity in the setting of atopy, during the course of a typical allergic reaction, and in allergic asthma.

Immunoglobulin: A protein produced by the body's immune system as part of an immune response to an antigen. Antigens can be infectious agents, such as viruses, bacteria, and parasites, or other proteins. When immunoglobulins are synthesized in response to an infection, they play a defensive and protective role. Immunoglobulins are sometimes called *gamma globulins*, an older terminology. Immunoglobulins are of five classes: IgA, IgD, IgE, IgG, and IgM.

Immunologist: A specialist in the science of immunology, which is concerned with various phenomena of immunity, sensitivity, and allergy.

Immunotherapy: This is one of the three main therapeutic approaches to the management of allergic disorders. Various terms have been used to describe this form of therapy, including *desensitization* (which is a misnomer), *hyposensitization*, or, most commonly, *allergy shots*. Patients are given subcutaneous injections of the specific allergens responsible for their symptoms. The purpose of the treatment is to decrease or eliminate the patient's sensitivity by stimulating the production of a protective (blocking) IgG antibody. The average duration of successful therapy generally takes between 3 to 5 years.

Incidence: In medicine, refers to the number of new cases of a disease at any point in time. To say, for example, that the incidence of peanut allergy increased in a certain community in the year 2004 compared with the prior year, you would need to count the number of new cases of peanut allergy in the community that were diagnosed in 2003, and compare it with the number of new cases found in 2004.

Inflammation: A physiologic process that plays a very important role in asthma. Inflammation occurs as consequence of the release of chemicals called *inflammatory mediators* from specialized white blood cells. The release of these chemicals, which occurs most often as the result of an allergic reaction, has the potential to cause chronic changes within the tissues of organs such as the lung. Over time, inflammation has the potential to damage organs, thereby making them less capable of performing their normal functions.

Influenza: Refers both to the influenza virus and the infectious illness caused by that virus in humans. Influenza begins abruptly and is characterized by high fever, chills, aches, and exhaustion. The illness is preventable through vaccination.

Inspiration: The act of taking a breath of air into the lungs. The respiratory cycle has two parts: inspiration and expiration.

Inspiratory: Refers to breathing in.

Internist: A physician specialized in the nonsurgical medical care of adults.

In vitro: A term derived from the Latin meaning: "in glass." Refers to a process carried out outside of a living organism, in an man-made environment such as a test tube or culture medium for instance. Any test or experiment performed in a laboratory would be considered an *in vitro* test.

In vivo: A term derived from the Lain meaning "within a living being." Allergy tests performed by prick/puncture or intradermal technique on a patient are *in vivo* procedures.

L

Larynx: The voice box. Two vocal cords allow for speech as inhaled air passes between them and creates vibrations within the larynx located in the mid-neck.

Leukotriene: Leukotrienes are inflammatory molecules. There are two families of leukotrienes. One in particular, called the *cysteinyl-leukotriene*, is important in asthma and allergy. Cysteinyl-leukotrienes are released in increased numbers during asthma exacerbations. Drugs, known as *leukotriene modifiers* have been developed based on current knowledge of leukotrienes. The leukotriene modifiers include (1) receptor antagonists or blockers, and (2) synthesis inhibitors. The first class blocks the effects of leukotrienes (blockers), whereas the second interferes with their formation (synthesis inhibitors). Medicines in the first category are very safe and widely used in the maintenance treatment of allergic rhinitis and asthma.

M

Mediator: Chemical compounds that are either preformed or actively produced by specialized white blood cells as the result of an allergic reaction. These substances are responsible for the rapid onset of symptoms such as sneeze, runny nose, tearing eyes, cough, and wheeze, and the delayed development of inflammation.

Metered-dose inhaler (MDI): A device that allows the delivery of a precise and accurate dose of medicine to the lungs through inhalation. MDIs are reliable, portable, and very convenient. Many different types of respiratory medicines come in MDI form, including short-acting bronchodilators, inhaled steroids, and anti-inflammatory medicines, as well as inhaled anticholinergics. Medicines in MDI form are used to treat asthma and chronic obstructive pulmonary disease. The newer MDIs use a chlorofluorocarbon-free propellant, usually hydrofluoroalkane.

Methacholine challenge test: The methacholine challenge test is a type of bronchoprovocation test. It is a specialized pulmonary function test used in evaluating suspected asthma when the diagnosis is otherwise uncertain. Methacholine challenge testing can identify bronchial hyperresponsiveness.

Molecular biology: The study of the structure, function, and reactions of DNA, RNA, proteins, and other molecules involved in the life processes.

Morbidity: A measure of illness in a given population. The yearly morbidity rate from a disease is defined as the proportion of people affected by that disease per year, per given unit of population.

Mortality: A measure of illness based on the rate of death from a disease in a given community or population at a precise point in time. The yearly mortality rate from a disease is defined as the ratio of deaths caused by that disease to the total number of persons in that community or population.

Mucus: Mucus is a mixture composed of water, salt, and proteins produced by specialized cells in the nose, sinuses, and lung passages. Mucus plays a defensive role and helps to protect from infection. Mucus is also produced in increased quantities as a consequence of irritation of the mucus-producing glands, as often occurs transiently in asthma exacerbations and on a more long-term basis in chronic smokers. Doctors often use the phrase *mucus hypersecretion* when extra mucus develops.

N

National Asthma Education and Prevention Program (NAEPP): The NAEPP was founded in 1989 under the auspices of the National Institute of Health's National Heart, Lung, and Blood Institute. The NAEPP aims to improve asthma care in the United States by teaching health professionals, asthma patients, and the general public about asthma. The NEAPP's panel of experts has published several expert panel reports with guidelines for the diagnosis and management of asthma.

Nebulizer: A device that transforms a respiratory drug in liquid form into a fine mist of medicine particles that are easily inhaled into the respiratory passages. It is powered by a machine or compressor that uses electrical current or batteries. Nebulizers are used for treatment in babies and very young children with asthma who cannot use an MDI or DPI. They are also often used in an emergency setting. Several different classes of asthma medicines are available for nebulization, including β_2 agonists and inhaled corticosteroid preparations.

Nocturnal: Taking place or occurring during the nighttime. Asthmatic exacerbations, for example, usually include nocturnal symptoms.

O

Obesity: Obesity refers to the condition of being significantly overweight or obese. Persons are obese if they weigh more than 30% above their ideal body weight for their given age, height, and gender. Another definition of obesity involves computation of the BMI. An overweight adult has a BMI of between 25 and 30, whereas an obese adult has a BMI of 30 or greater.

Obstructive dysfunction: A pattern of abnormality detected through pulmonary function testing. Several different lung conditions lead to obstructive dysfunction on spirometry, one of the pulmonary function tests. Asthma is one of the conditions that, on testing, demonstrates obstructive dysfunction. A key element of the obstructive dysfunction uniquely seen in asthma is that, by definition, the obstruction (or abnormality) is completely reversible.

Oral: By mouth. Oral medications are taken by mouth and swallowed. Once swallowed, they dissolve in the digestive tract and become absorbed into the bloodstream. From there, they enter the organs and tissues to exert their pharmacologic effects. Oral medicines come in tablet, capsule, chewable, and liquid forms.

Otorhinolaryngologist: A specialist in diseases involving the ears, nose, and throat. Commonly referred to as an ENT specialist.

Oxygen (O$_2$): An odorless, colorless gas necessary for life. The air we breathe is composed of 21% oxygen.

P

Pathologic: Abnormal finding or feature indicative of the presence of a medical condition or disease. A cough, for example, is not normal, and when present in a child is considered pathological from a medical perspective. The science that studies the causes and the nature of diseases is the science of pathology.

Peak Expiratory Flow (PEF): The PEF is part of the several different measurements obtained during the spirometry portion of PFTs. Because exacerbations of asthma lead to decreasing values of PEF, self-monitoring at home of PEF in asthma is part of contemporary asthma management. Measuring PEF helps guide therapy. If the PEF begins to drop, individuals with asthma may need to restart their fast-acting, quick-relief inhaler and increase their dose of inhaled corticosteroid, for example. Lightweight, home peak flow monitors are convenient and easy to use, even by children.

Pediatrician: A medical specialist who has received intensive training in the care and treatment of children from birth to young adulthood.

Percussion: A technique used during the physical examination of the lungs that consists of tapping gently on the chest wall and listening to the quality of the sound produced. Healthy air-filled lungs are resonant to percussion. Pneumonia or a fluid collection around the lungs, on the other hand, gives rise to dullness to percussion.

Pharmacotherapy: Treatment by medication administered either by mouth, through injection, or intravenously.

Postnatally: After birth. Human lungs continue to grow and develop postnatally, after birth and into infancy.

Prevalence: In medicine, the total number of cases of a disease diagnosed at a given point in time. It includes all cases, whether the diagnosis is new or longstanding. To assess the prevalence of asthma in a community as of January 1, for example, you would count all persons who were ever told by a medical professional that they had a diagnosis of asthma.

Puberty: The time during which sexual maturation begins. Also refers to the time when reproductive organs develop to allow reproduction.

Pulmonary Function Tests (PFTs): Include the measurement of lung volumes, spirometry, diffusion, and sometimes arterial blood gasses.

Pulmonary symptomatology: Symptoms related to the lungs and the act of breathing. Wheezing, cough, breathlessness, and mucus production are examples of pulmonary symptomatology.

Pulmonologist: A physician specialist with extra training and qualifications in the diagnosis and treatment of lung diseases. Some pulmonologists are also pediatric specialists and are known as *pediatric pulmonologists.* Pediatric pulmonologists treat babies, children, and adolescents with lung diseases. Adult pulmonologists are internists with additional specialty training who limit their practice to adults with respiratory conditions.

R

RAST®: RAST® is an abbreviation for *RadioAllergoSorbentTest*, a trademark of Pharmacia Diagnostics that originated and developed the first RAST® test. RAST® is a laboratory allergy test that detects and measures the level of IgE antibodies directed against specific antigens in a blood sample. Measuring blood RAST® is one way of assessing the possible presence of an allergy. If a person is suspected of being allergic to grass, for example, his or her doctor might send a blood sample for RAST® testing. The doctor would request a test that would detect significant levels of IgE directed against grasses. The absence of any detectable IgE to grasses would argue against a grass allergy.

Reflux: A backward flow. Gastric fluid moving up into the esophagus from the stomach is referred to as *gastroesophageal reflux.*

Refractory: Resistant to treatment.

Rhinosinusitis: Refers to an inflammatory process or disease state involving the nasal and sinus passages. *See also* rhinitis and sinusitis.

Remission: When used in a medical context, a remission refers to the subsiding of disease symptoms. A person with asthma who enters a period in which no asthma symptoms are experienced has entered a period of asthma remission. The disease is still present, but is quiescent because it has no symptoms.

Remodeling: Irreversible and permanent (anatomic and functional) changes that can occur in an asthmatic's lungs over time, thought to be a result of uncontrolled and untreated lung inflammation.

Respiration: Refers to the act of breathing in (inspiration) and then out (expiration). Also refers to the process whereby the lungs exchange gases, more specifically, oxygen and carbon dioxide at the level of the alveolus and the alveolar-capillary membrane.

Respiratory failure: A state or illness in which the lungs become incapable of respiration. They become unable to provide the body with needed oxygen, and cannot rid the body of accumulated carbon dioxide and metabolic waste products. Respiratory failure can be acute, as after a major trauma such as a car accident, for example, or chronic, as in the case of emphysema. Uncontrolled asthma can result in progressive respiratory failure, which is a true medical emergency. When untreated, respiratory failure is fatal.

Respiratory rate: Number of breaths per minute.

Retractions: A "sucking in" or visible depression of the muscles in the spaces between the ribs that occurs with labored breathing.

Rhinitis: An inflammation involving the mucous membranes of the nose. Rhinitis may be allergic or nonallergic. Allergic rhinitis may be seasonal, occurring only in spring, or perennial, with symptoms that are present throughout the year. Typical examples of seasonal rhinitis include ragweed pollen allergy (hay fever) and tree or grass pollen allergy (rose fever). Perennial rhinitis symptoms may occur because of sensitivity to dust mites or a household pet. Typical symptoms include sneeze, runny nose, nasal congestion, and tearing and itching of the eyes.

S

Sensitization: In the context of allergies, sensitization is the process by which a person becomes, over time, increasingly allergic to a substance (sensitizer) through repeated exposure to that substance.

Sensitizer: A substance that causes an allergic response in a child who has become "sensitized" to that specific substance by a previous exposure or multiple past exposures.

Sinus: The sinuses are air-filled cavities within the human skull. Adults have several sinuses, named by location: the frontal, ethmoid, sphenoid, and maxillary sinuses. The sinuses continue to form after birth; consequently, the fron-

tal and sphenoid sinuses are not well developed in children.

Sinusitis: An inflammation of the lining of sinuses caused most commonly by either infection (viral or bacterial sinusitis) or allergy (allergic sinusitis).

Spacer: A device that facilitates the inhalation of medicine from a metered-dose inhaler (MDI). Different brands and designs of spacers are available. Spacers allow one to space the required steps for correct MDI use over time. Correct MDI technique requires the user to simultaneously activate the MDI canister, release the medicine, and inhale as deeply as possible. Adding a spacer permits the user to first activate the medicine and then inhale deeply. Spacers make it easier to use the MDI medicine, enhance medication delivery to the lungs, and reduce deposition of medicine on the voice box. The last fact is important because deposition of inhaler medicine in the throat and on the vocal cords not only wastes medicine but also can lead to throat irritation and hoarseness. Holding chambers are one type of spacer devices; some people use the terms interchangeably.

Spirometry: Spirometry is a pulmonary function test (PFT) and is the most important PFT in diagnosing and treating asthma. Spirometry measures the flow of air from the lungs as a person forcefully and fully exhales from a deep inspiration. During the performance of spirometry, a subject is first asked to take in a very deep breath, and then blow it out as hard and as quickly as possible. Spirometry is used to detect the presence of obstructive dysfunction. If obstructive dysfunction is, in fact, present, spirometry also measures the extent of the dysfunction. An individual with well-controlled and asymptomatic asthma usually has normal values on spirometry. An exacerbation of asthma will cause the emergence of an obstructive dysfunction pattern on spirometry.

Steroids: *See* corticosteroids.

Stethoscope: A medical instrument used to amplify and listen to sounds produced by internal organs, such as the lungs, heart, or bowels, during a physical examination. The process of listening through the stethoscope is called auscultation. The French physician René Laënnec (1781–1826) is credited with the invention of the stethoscope.

Symptoms: Abnormal feelings, occurrences, or functions that differ from usual. Symptoms are noticed and experienced by the patient who would then report them to their treating physician. Symptoms can relate to changes in body appearance, function, or sensations. Symptoms are, by definition, subjective. A physician can inquire about the presence, absence, or intensity of a symptom, but cannot by definition detect it on a physical examination or on a lab test Examples of symptoms include pain, breathlessness, chest tightness, and fatigue.

T

Trachea: The scientific name for the windpipe. The uppermost portion of the trachea can be felt in the front of the neck. The trachea leads air from the back of the nose and throat into the lungs.

Tracheomalacia: A self-correcting condition found in some newborns caused by immature development of the cartilaginous rings that provide the framework for the trachea.

Trigger: In the context of asthma, a trigger is a stimulus to asthma or allergy. For example, asthma symptoms may worsen when an individual with asthma is ill with a viral respiratory infection. In that situation, the infection is considered a trigger for worsening asthma. Similarly, a person who is allergic to cats will notice itchy eyes and a runny nose triggered by entering a room with a resident cat. Part of allergy and asthma treatment involves correct identification of symptom triggers, with the goal of avoiding them as much as possible.

U

Urticaria: Urticaria is the scientific name for hives, a type of skin rash. Hives, or urticaria, are raised, welt-like, reddened, and intensely itchy. The most common cause of urticaria is an allergic reaction. Sometimes, urticaria are idiopathic, meaning that no cause can be identified. Urticaria are treated with anti-inflammatory agents or antihistamines, or both.

V

Vaccine: A vaccine is a specialized preparation designed to stimulate the body's immune system to make protective antibodies directed against a specific infectious agent. Some vaccines are injected into muscle or skin, whereas others are inhaled or swallowed. Some vaccines protect against specific viruses, such as influenza or polio; others protect against bacteria, such as haemophilus (HiB) or pneumococcus. Some vaccines contain a live, weakened strain, whereas others contain only a portion of the infectious agent.

Vocal Cord Dysfunction Syndrome (VCD): A condition that can be confused with asthma. VCD's primary disturbance involves the vocal cords and their abnormal tendency to move toward each other (rather than move apart) during inspiration, or breathing in. It is important to diagnose VCD if it is present, because asthma treatments will not be effective for VCD.

Viral: Caused by or related to a virus.

Virus: A type of infectious agent. Viruses contain a single strand of either DNA or RNA, surrounded by a protein coat. Because they only contain one strand of genetic information, viruses cannot replicate on their own and require a host cell for replication. Different viruses have different degrees of infectivity and also infect different species. Some viruses infect plants, for example. Viruses that infect humans can cause disease. Depending on the particular virus and the underlying health of the human, viral infections can run the gamut from mild to life-threatening. Influenza virus, for example, can be fatal.

W

Wheeze: The typical sound associated with asthma. It has been described as a rattling or whistling noise heard primarily when a child breathes out (exhales). This sound develops because of narrowing or constriction of the bronchial passageways and the accumulation of thickened mucous secretions within the bronchial passages.

Index